SpringerBriefs in Psychology

SpringerBriefs present concise summaries of cutting-edge research and practical applications across a wide spectrum of fields. Featuring compact volumes of 50 to 125 pages, the series covers a range of content from professional to academic. Typical topics might include:

- A timely report of state-of-the-art analytical techniques
- A bridge between new research results as published in journal articles and a contextual literature review
- A snapshot of a hot or emerging topic
- An in-depth case study or clinical example
- A presentation of core concepts that readers must understand to make independent contributions

SpringerBriefs in Psychology showcase emerging theory, empirical research, and practical application in a wide variety of topics in psychology and related fields. Briefs are characterized by fast, global electronic dissemination, standard publishing contracts, standardized manuscript preparation and formatting guidelines, and expedited production schedules.

More information about this series at http://www.springer.com/series/10143

Yara Nico · Jan Luiz Leonardi ·
Larissa Zeggio

Depression as a Cultural Phenomenon in Postmodern Society

An Analytical-Behavioral Essay of Our Time

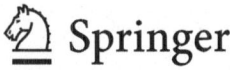 Springer

Yara Nico
São Paulo, Brazil

Larissa Zeggio
Instituto Brasileiro de Inteligência
Emocional e Social (IBIES)
Florianópolis, Santa Catarina, Brazil

Jan Luiz Leonardi
Instituto de Psicologia
Baseada em Evidências
São Paulo, Brazil

ISSN 2192-8363   ISSN 2192-8371   (electronic)
SpringerBriefs in Psychology
ISBN 978-3-030-60544-5   ISBN 978-3-030-60545-2   (eBook)
https://doi.org/10.1007/978-3-030-60545-2

Foreword

Popular culture says that depression is contained anger. I think everyone who has experienced depression, from mild to severe forms, will understand that statement and agree with it...

It is also true that when one looks around, it is very easy to find a person who suffers in a way that we could call "depressed." This problem is so common that it has become part of our daily lives and has brought the word depression into the lay language. People often want to express sadness or discouragement—or even just tiredness—but end up using "depressed," a technical term from health sciences.

To clarify these issues, the book *Depression as a Cultural Phenomenon in Postmodern Society* brings us an in-depth analysis of the clinical phenomenon technically called depression—or more specifically "Major Depressive Disorder"—in a way that interests both health professionals and lay persons.

This book interests everyone because it broadly addresses the phenomenon of depression. From its origins as a scientific concept to its sociological explanations to expounding its emergence, the book presents in a very well-founded way, in a scientifically grounded way, the knowledge necessary to clarify, understand, and seek treatment and prevention for this major social evil.

The authors began this work with a description of the current diagnostic parameters of MDD followed by alarming global epidemiological data showing that depression has affected all races, social classes, genders, and creeds. They then address the topic departing from an approach based on the behavior analysis, laying the foundations for the compilation of factors that could contribute to the emergence of a defined outline of depression. This is where the book takes an even greater leap and gains amplitude: besides analyzing proposals of great radical behaviorist authors, Yara Nico, Jan Leonardi, and Larissa Zeggio highlight other explanations based on solid data from diverse experimental models, establishing a dialogue that removes analysts from their conceptual and theoretical entrenchment. They establish connections with the respect that other professionals deserve, and they have as a first result a clarifying panorama from the peculiar vision with which behavioral analysis contributes to reduce the suffering of individuals.

The authors emphasized the role of verbal behavior as one of the determinants of the depressive process. This work values all the development of research on this subject and consolidates technical approaches that help in the treatment of depression.

The dialogue continues in the third part of the book with philosophical and conceptual interpretations that differ from those of behavior analysis. It confronts sociological and cultural development approaches with an alarming picture in which social relationships are broken up. At this point, the profound social changes needed to prevent depression from spreading are revealed and pointed out. Once again, exponents of behavioral analysis have their ideas represented together with those of other postmodern historians and sociologists on the analysis of depression. The result is coherent and indicative of new factors contributing to the determination of and the need for social change.

For all these reasons, *Depression as a Cultural Phenomenon in Postmodern Society* is a necessary book. It helps to raise awareness of the gravity and depth of the problem, modulates our behavior in ways different from those we have practiced, and points out ways to confront the problem, whether it is already present or needs to be eliminated before it even manifests.

São Paulo, Brazil   Roberto Alves Banaco

Contents

About the Authors

Yara Nico is a Clinical Psychologist with a degree in Psychology from the Pontifical Catholic University of São Paulo (PUC-SP), Brazil, and a Master's degree in Experimental Psychology: Behavior Analysis from the same institution. She has more than 20 years of experience as a therapist and a teacher in higher education. She has developed the pedagogical project and the curriculum framework for the Centro Universitário Nove de Julho Psychology Department. She implemented and was responsible for the general coordination of this department (2001–2006), where she also worked as a professor. She was a professor at PUC-SP and at Universidade São Judas Tadeu. She was the pedagogical coordinator of the specialization course in Analytical-Behavioral Therapy at the Núcleo Paradigma de Análise do Comportamento (2007–2014). As a researcher, she works mainly on the Theory of Relational Mouldings (RFT) and Cultural Determinants of Contemporary Psychological Suffering.

Jan Luiz Leonardi has a degree in Psychology from the Pontifical Catholic University of São Paulo (PUC-SP), Brazil; specialization in Behavior Therapy from Paradigma—Centro de Ciências e Tecnologia do Comportamento, intensive training in Dialectical Behavior Therapy from Behavioral Tech, a master's degree in Experimental Psychology: Behavior Analysis from PUC-SP and a doctorate in Clinical Psychology from the University of São Paulo (USP), Brazil. He is currently the coordinator of the Evidence-Based Psychotherapy Training at InPBE—Institute for Evidence-Based Practice in Psychology and a professor in Paradigma, in addition to working as a clinical psychologist.

Larissa Zeggio is a Psychotherapist at Clínica Mudanças Positivas in Florianópolis, Brazil. She holds a degree in Clinical Psychology from Faculdade Paulistana de Ciências e Letras (FAPA), Brazil, a master's degree in Health Sciences (Psychobiology) from the Federal University of São Paulo (UNIFESP), Brazil, a doctorate in Sciences-Neurosciences from UNIFESP, a postdoctorate in Cognition from UNIFESP, and is currently a postdoctorate fellow in Education at the Federal University of Paraná (UFPR), Brazil. She has 18 years of experience in teaching higher education, graduate and postgraduate courses, in supervising studies in psychology, coordinating training courses for professionals in Health and Education. Founder of R-Club, a social network platform to spread resilience and emotional intelligence [https://resilienciaclub.com/]. Currently, she is a member of the Board of Directors of the Brazilian Institute of Social and Emotional Intelligence (IBIES), Technical Coordinator of the FRIENDS Method in Brazil, Coordinator of the specialization course in Clinical Neuropsychology, and guest professor for the Centro Sul Brasileiro de Pesquisa, Extensão e Pós-Graduação (CENSUPEG) postgraduate course, and a Clinical Psychologist. She is the local coordinator of Pint of Science (Florianópolis) and coorganizer of "Neuromyths busters" that discusses prevention in mental health and neuroscience. Researcher in of Neuroscience and Psychology, working mainly on learning and emotional memory, neuropsychology, social-emotional skills, prevention and promotion in mental health, neuroscience and education, and scientific dissemination.

Chapter 1
Introduction

Major Depressive Disorder (MDD), often simply called depression, is character-ized by sadness, loss of the ability to feel pleasure, lack of interest, feeling of uselessness, excessive guilt, fatigue, difficulty concentrating, psychomotor retarda-tion, insomnia or hypersomnia, among others, and it is responsible for clinically significant suffering and impairment of functioning in important areas of life (Moreno et al. 2007, 2012). The DSM-5, the latest edition of the *Diagnostic and Statistical Manual of Mental Disorders* (American Psychiatric Association 2013), presents the following diagnostic criteria for MDD:

A. Five (or more) of the following symptoms were present during 2 consecutive weeks and represented a change in relation to the previous functioning; at least one of the symptoms is: (1) depressed mood or (2) loss of interest or pleasure.

   1. Depressed mood most of the day, almost every day, as indicated by a subjec-tive story (e.g., feel sad, empty, without hope) or by observation made by other people (e.g., it seems funny).
   2. Accentuated decrease of interest or pleasure in all or almost all activities most of the day, almost every day (indicated by subjective story or observation made by other people).
   3. Loss or significant weight gain without dieting (e.g., an alteration of more than 5% of body weight in one month), or reduction or increase in appetite almost every day.
   4. Insomnia or hypersomnia almost every day.
   5. Agitation or psychomotor retardation almost every day (observed by other people, not merely subjective feelings of restlessness or being slowed down).
   6. Fatigue or loss of energy almost every day.
   7. Daily feelings of uselessness or excessive or inappropriate guilt (which may be delusional and not merely self-recrimination or guilt of being sick).
   8. Reduced ability to think or concentrate, or indecision almost every day (through subjective report or observation by other people).

1

Y. Nico et al., *Depression as a Cultural Phenomenon in Postmodern Society*,
SpringerBriefs in Psychology, https://doi.org/10.1007/978-3-030-60545-2_1

9. Recurring thoughts of death (not just dying), recurring suicidal ideation without a specific plane, an attempt to commit suicide or a specific plane to commit suicide.

B. The symptoms cause clinically significant suffering or prejudice in the social, professional, or other important areas of the individual's life.

C. The episode is not attributable to the physiological effects of a substance or to another general medical condition (e.g., hypothyroidism).

D. The occurrence of a major depressive episode is not better explained by schizoaffective disorder, schizophrenia, schizophreniform disorder, delusional disorder, other schizophrenia spectrum disorders, other specified psychotic disorders, schizophrenia disorders, or other unspecified psychotic disorders.

E. There was never a manic episode or a hypomanic episode.

The epidemiology of depression is alarming. Recent research (World Health Organization [WHO] 2017) indicates that more than 300 million people in the world are undergoing diagnostic tests for MDD. For this reason, MDD was the only psychiatric condition included in the *World Health Survey*. This study was carried out at the beginning of the twenty-first century by the WHO in 60 countries to assess the prevalence and degree of commitment to a wide range of health problems (Kessler 2012).

In 2008, WHO published the results of a more specific work on the subject— a *World Research on Mental Health*. This is a set of epidemiological research on psychiatric disorders carried out in 18 countries across all continents. Ten developed countries (Germany, Belgium, Spain, France, Holland, Italy, Israel, Japan, New Zealand, and USA) and eight developing countries (Brazil, Colombia, Mexico, Ukraine, Lebanon, India, South Africa, and China) participated in this research. By means of a standardized instrument capable of detecting different DSM-IV-TR diagnoses, researches assessed prevalence rates, age of onset, disease course, sociodemographic correlates, and treatments (Kessler and Üstün 2008).

The data showed that the prevalence of MDD over the life span differs considerably between countries, generally being higher in developed countries than in developing countries. The lowest prevalence of MDD was 6.6% (Japan) and the highest was 19.2% (USA). On the other hand, the prevalence in the 12 months prior to the survey was higher in developing countries, reaching the highest rate in São Paulo, Brazil (Kessler and Üstün 2008; Kessler and Bromet 2013). In addition, data from 18 countries revealed that 40% of individuals had their first episode of depression within 20 years, 50% between 20 and 50 years, and only 10% after 65 years (Kessler et al. 2010). Other studies (e.g., Birmaher et al. 2004) showed that the prevalence of MDD is 1% in preschool children, 2% in school-age children, and 5–8% in adolescents. In terms of gender, women have two to three times greater chance of developing depression than men.

Several sociodemographic factors are correlated to an increased risk of developing depression, namely: living traumatic experiences in childhood, such as negligence; divorce or death of a parent; physical, emotional or sexual abuse; living with family members who are depressed; losing a spouse due to divorce or death; being forever lost; etc. (Kessler and Bromet 2013; Bonde 2008; Kessler 1997) and social inequality (Hidaka 2012).

Data collected from the *World Research on Mental Health* revealed that a significant proportion of individuals diagnosed with MDD remain untreated. In developed countries, 35.5–50.3% of serious cases did not receive any type of intervention in the 12 months prior to the survey, and in developing countries, this number reached 85.4% (The WHO World Mental Health Survey Consortium 2004). This is a worrisome trend, since, in addition to depression, it is estimated that 15% of depressed people suffer suicide (Chachamovich et al. 2009). Among individuals who seek treatment, a significant proportion presents a chronic condition with many relapses (Hardeveld et al. 2010; Clumsy and Klein 2008).

Another study that highlights the commitment caused by depression is the *Global Burden of Diseases, Injuries, and Risk Factors Study* (GBD), which consists of a set of researches carried out by the WHO in partnership with six universities in the USA, England, Australia, and Japan, with editions in 1990, 2000, and 2010 (Murray et al. 2012a, b). The objective of these studies was to quantify the impact of 291 health problems, considering 67 risk factors and 1,160 sequels. For this purpose, a unified method was created, capable of measuring and comparing the damages brought about by the different conditions in the two categories: (1) years of life lost, which refers to the premature mortality attributable to the disease; (2) years lived with incapacitation, which refers to the period of time in which the individual has significant impairments in his personal, social, occupational, etc., life as a result of the clinical condition he presents (Murray et al. 2012c; You et al. 2012). Ferrari et al. (2013) reviewed the epidemiological studies that made up the 2010 GBD and found that the highest rate of "years of life lost" was in Africa, followed by Iraq, with the lowest being in Japan (Ferrari et al. 2013). The methodology employed by Ferrari et al. (2013) was able to capture data on the prevalence of countries in conflict, such as Afghanistan and Iraq. In the case of North Africa and the Middle East, the conflict in the region increased the position of the MDD in the GBD ranking, being associated with risk factors such as conflict, child sexual abuse and violence by intimate partners (Ferrari et al. 2013).

An example of incapacitation associated with depression is the reduction of productivity at work, which, in some cases, can lead to unemployment (Lépine and Briley 2011). A study carried out in the USA (Bromet et al. 2011) revealed that, on average, 27.2 days of work per year were wasted by each depressed individual, considering both absenteeism (temporary absence from work due to illness) and presence (being physically present in the work environment, but presenting little or no performance). These lost days represented, on average, a loss of $4,400 dollars per year for each depressed individual, totaling $36.6 billion dollars in the year. Other examples of incapacitation associated with depression include dropping out of school, problems in married life, bad parenting, among others (Kessler 2012; Kessler and Bromet 2013; Lépine and Briley 2011).

Through the two measures described above (years of life lost and years lived with incapacitation), MDD was classified in the 1990 GBD as the fourth leading disease responsible for the loss of 1 year of a healthy life. It then moved into third place in the 2000 GBD and reached second place in the 2010 GBD, a trend that may indicate an increase in cases of depression. In fact, it is estimated that depression will be the main cause of incapacitation in 2030 (Brometet al. 2011; Lépine and Briley 2011). But, modern times have struck hard and brought about this reality sooner: in November 2014, the seminar, *The Global Crisis of Depression*, promoted by the magazine *The Economist,* began with the news that depression is now the most incapacitating disease. In the words of Hidaka: "the evidence suggests that we may indeed be in the midst of an epidemic of depression" (Hidaka 2012). In this sense, it is worth noting that, in 2010, the direct and indirect costs of depression worldwide were around $800 billion dollars, and it is estimated that this amount will be more than double in the next 20 years. Currently, indirect costs (e.g., days lost in productivity due to absenteeism) are responsible for 63% of the total cost of depression, while approximately 1% refers to the cost of psychotherapy and 3.5% to medication.

The numbers shown by the epidemiological researches allow us to affirm that depressive symptoms can be understood as a contemporary form of malaise; as a species of suffering that current culture produces in its individuals. There are several complex social contingencies in the contemporary world responsible for a high number of people presenting a similar behavioral pattern, which are called depression. When an operant behavior is independently emitted by many people, but with a similar effect on the world, we say that it is a cultural practice. Therefore, it is possible to state that the set of behaviors that compose the diagnosis of depression consists of cultural practice in the present world. The cumulative and measurable effects of a cultural practice can be beneficial or harmful to the social cohesion and general well-being of the members of a society (Biglan and Glenn 2013). There is no doubt that the effects of depression, as a cultural practice of the present time, have been harmful and of great magnitude not only for depressed individuals and their families but also for society in general. The cumulative effects on the well-being of a significant number of people make this cultural practice a social issue (Malagodi and Jackson 1989) and, in the case of depression, a public health problem.

It is already considered cliché to say that the world is no longer the same, that social relations are changing at an unprecedented speed, and that we live in a world of unfrequented consumption and without utopias. Without wanting to retell this often-told tale, and without the ambition of exaggerating the understanding of what defines social life in our time, the present work intends to offer a characterization of contemporary society so that, based on the experimental and interpretative models produced by Behavior Analysis, we can think about how the social contingencies of our times can affect the lives of individuals in the most depressing way. In addition, the identification of cultural practices related to depression in the world today will be, in this book, a starting point for thinking about the organization of social contingencies of reinforcement that produce and sustain operant behaviors with beneficial effects for society in general and for individuals in particular. Innovative proposals and evidence of results of programs that manage social contingencies to prevent depression and promote well-being will be presented in the second part of this book.

A brief overview of the existing models of Behavioral Analysis for the understanding of depressive patterns will be presented, followed by a characterization of premodern, modern, and postmodern societies with the aim of highlighting some factors related to the production of depression as a cultural phenomenon today.

References

American Psychiatric Association. (2013). *Diagnostic and statistical manual of mental disorders: DSM-5*. Arlington: American Psychiatric Publishing.

Biglan, A., & Glenn, S. S. (2013). Toward prosocial behavior and environments: Behavioral and cultural contingencies in a public health framework.

Birmaher, B., Williamson, D. E., Dahl, R. E., Axelson, D. A., Kaufman, J., Dorn, L. D., et al. (2004). Clinical presentation and course of depression in youth: Does onset in childhood differ from onset in adolescence? *Journal of the American Academy of Child and Adolescent Psychiatry, 43*, 63–70.

Bonde, J. P. (2008). Psychosocial factors at work and risk of depression: A systematic review of the epidemiological evidence. *Journal of Occupational and Environmental Medicine, 65*, 438–445.

Bromet, E., Andrade, L. H., Hwang, I., Sampson, N. A., Alonso, J., Girolamo, G., et al. (2011). Cross-national epidemiology of DSM-IV major depressive episode. *BMC Medicine, 9*, 90.

Chachamovich, E., Stefanello, S., Botega, N., & Turecki, G. (2009). What are the recent clinical findings on the association between depression and suicide? *Brazilian Journal of Psychiatry, 31*, 518–525.

Clumsy, D. C., & Klein, D. N. (2008). Chronic depression: Update on classification and treatment. *Current Psychiatry Reports, 10*, 458–464.

Ferrari, A. J., Charlson, F. J., Norman, R. E., Patten, S. B., Freedman, G., Murray, C. J., et al. (2013). Burden of depressive disorders by country, sex, age, and year: Findings from the global burden of disease study 2010. *PLoS Med, 10*(11), e1001547.

Hardeveld, F., Spijker, J., De Graaf, R., Nolen, W. A., & Beekman, A. T. (2010). Prevalence and predictors of recurrence of major depressive disorder in the adult population. *Scandinavian Psychiatric Act, 22*, 184–191.

Hidaka. (2012). Depression as a disease of modernity: Explanations for increasing prevalence. *Journal of Affective Disorders, 140*, 205–214.

Kessler, R. C. (1997). The effects of stressful life events on depression. *Annual Review of Psychology, 48*, 191–214.

Kessler, R. C. (2012). The costs of depression. *Psychiatric Clinics of North America, 35*, 1–14.

Kessler, R. C., Birnbaum, H., Shahly, V., Bromet, E., Hwang, I., McLaughlin, K. A., et al. (2010). Age differences in the prevalence and comorbidity of DSM-IV major depressive episodes: Results from the WHO world mental health survey initiative. *Depression and Anxiety, 27*, 351–364.

Kessler, R. C., & Bromet, E. J. (2013). The epidemiology of depression across cultures. *Annual Review of Public Health, 34*, 119–138.

Kessler, R. C., & Üstün, T. B. (2008). *The WHO world mental health surveys: Global perspectives on the epidemiology of mental disorders*. New York, NY: Cambridge University Press.

Lépine, J. P., & Briley. (2011). The increasing burden of depression. *Neuropsychiatric Disease and Treatment, 7*, 3–7.

Malagodi, E. F., & Jackson, K. (1989). Behavior analysts and cultural analysis: Troubleshooting and issues. *The Behavior Analyst, 12*(1), 17.

Moreno, D. H., Dias, R. S., & Moreno, R. A. (2007). Mood disorders. In M. R. Louzã Neto & H. Elkis (Eds.), *Basic psychiatry* (2nd ed., pp. 219–234). Porto Alegre, RS: Artmed.

Moreno, D. H., Moreno, R. A., & Soeiro-de-Souza, M. G. (2012). Disordered depression over the course of a lifetime. In O. V. Forlenza & E. C. Miguel (Eds.), *Compêndio de clinicapsiquiátrica* (pp. 296–314). Barueri, SP: Manole.

Murray, C. J. L., Ezzati, M., Flaxman, A. D., Lim, S., Lozano, R., Michaud, C., et al. (2012a). GBD 2010: A multi-investigator collaboration for global comparative descriptive epidemiology. *The Lancet, 380*(15), 2055–2058.

Murray, C. J. L, Ezzati, M., Flaxman, A. D., Lim, S., Lozano, R., Michaud, C., et al. (2012b). GBD 2010: Design, definitions, and metrics. *The Lancet, 380*(25), 2063–2066.

Murray, C. J. L., Vos, T., Lozano, R., Naghavi, M., Flaxman, A. D., Michaud, C., et al. (2012c). Disability-adjusted life years (DALYs) for 291 diseases and injuries in 21 regions, 1990–2010: A systematic analysis for the Global Burden of Disease Study 2010. *The Lancet, 380*, 2197–2223.

The WHO World Mental Health Survey Consortium. (2004). Prevalence, severity, and unmet need for treatment of mental disorders in the World Health Organization World Mental Health Surveys. *Journal of the American Medical Association, 291*, 2581–2590.

World Health Organization (2017). Depression and other common mental disorders: global health estimates. Rep. CC BY-NC-SA 3.0 IGO. Geneva: World Health Organization.

You, T., Flaxman, A.D., Naghavi, M., Lozano, R., Michaud, C., Ezzati, M., et al. (2012). Years lived with disability (YLDs) for 1160 sequelae of 289 diseases and injuries 1990–2010: A systematic analysis for the global burden of disease study 2010. *The Lancet, 380*, 2163–2196.

Chapter 2
Behavior Analysis and Depression: Conceptual and Empirical Aspects

In 1973, Ferster (1973) proposed a behavior analytic interpretation for the phenomenon of depression (Ferster 1973). Based on the knowledge of the basic behavioral processes discovered by means of experimental studies, the author argued that the low density of positive reinforcing stimuli would be responsible for the central characteristics of MDD diagnosis. Symptoms described as lack of interest, fatigue and psychomotor retardation (i.e., low behavior) could be understood as a decrease in the individual's response due to the absence of positive reinforcement. In addition, symptoms such as sadness and incapacity to feel pleasure could also be explained according to this perspective, since the presentation of such stimuli generally elicits bodily sensations described as "pleasant" (Skinner 1976, especially Chap. 4). Ferster also suggested that much of the depressed individual's repertoire has an escape or avoidance function (Ferster 1973). Behaviors such as spending the day in bed and making facial expressions of sadness could have the function of diminishing, eliminating, or avoiding aversive tasks. Two decades later, Biglan (1991) presented a set of studies that confirmed this second hypothesis of Ferster (Biglan 1991).

As presented above, Ferster's interpretation (Ferster 1973) postulates that the behavioral repertoire typically involved in depression consists of the reduction of response classes controlled by positive reinforcement associated with the increase in response classes controlled by negative reinforcement. It is important to recognize that these two forms of control are directly related. The low frequency of positively reinforced behavior may be due to the high frequency of escape and avoidance behavior, which makes it difficult to separate the control variables. For example, imagine a person who spends the entire day in bed and does not go to work in order to avoid a meeting in which he or she will probably be reprimanded. Going to bed avoids the aversive event (reprehension) but also prevents the individual from getting in contact with positive reinforcement contingencies that could contribute to the change of his depressive condition.

Later, Lewinsohn and collaborators (Lewinsohn 1974, 1975; Lewisohn and Libet 1972; Lewisohn et al. 1976) deepened Ferster's model (Ferster 1973), suggesting that the depressed pattern would be the result of a history of low-density positive reinforcers contingent on responses. In this sense, depression would not only be characterized by the existence of few reinforcers but also by the fact that they are not directly produced by the individual's actions. In addition, Lewinsohn and collaborators listed three ways in which there could be a low density of positive reinforcers: (1) loss of the function of stimulating positive reinforcers from some environmental events; (2) unavailability of reinforcers due to environmental changes; and (3) lack of efficient behavioral repertoire to produce reinforcers that are available in the environment.

More recently, other behavior analysts (e.g., Dougher and Hackbert 1994; Kanter et al. 2004, 2005, 2007, 2008) have revisited Ferster's and Lewinsohn's models and advanced the behavior analytic interpretation of depression. Kanter et al. (2005) suggested that the loss of the positive reinforcement stimulus function of some environmental events and the consequent decrease of several types of response could be due to the erosion of reinforcement, a process by which reinforcement stimuli cease to have this function over time through habituation or satiation. In this case, the events continue to be present in the individual's environment, but their reinforcing properties diminish or cease to exist (Kanter et al. 2005). For example, the reinforcing value of the sexual contact with a certain partner may diminish considerably after a long history of familiarity and routine in conjugal life. In a similar way, a friend's jokes, which are very funny in the first times, may become flat and tedious after some repetitions.

Although well known by behavioral analysts and implicit in Ferster's model (Ferster 1973), another process involving the decrease in positive reinforcement density mentioned by the authors (e.g., Dougher and Hackbert 1994; Kanter et al. 2005, 2008) is extinction, in which there is an abrupt rupture of a relationship already established between response and reinforcement that, in addition to making the operant in question weaker, produces feelings of frustration, incapacity, and revolt (Skinner 1965, 1976). In this case, therefore, the individual gives the answer, but the reinforcing consequence does not occur.

Kanter et al. (2005) also proposed that the decrease in response and the feeling of lack of will observed in the depressive condition may be the result of a history of intermittent reinforcement ratio, in which the demands for the liberation of the reformer become very high or increase rapidly, which is called ratio strain in the literature (Kanter et al. 2005, cf. Catania 1999). Experimental studies with laboratory animals (Ferster and Skinner 1957) have shown that the abrupt passage from a low ratio to a very high ratio ceases to respond and generates a state that could be described as apathy and exhaustion.

Another contingency that should be considered is the punishment. According to Dougher and Hackbert (Lewisohn et al. 1976), it is common for people with chronic depression to have gone through a long history of punishment. It is known that punishment produces some significant effects (Skinner 1965, 1991): (1) elicits incompatible responses with punished behavior, preventing it from occurring; (2) establishes the individual's own response as a source of aversive stimulation, leading to feelings of guilt typical of depressive condition; (3) leads the individual to do anything to reduce the aversive stimulation originated by their own behavior; (4) leads the individual to avoid contact with the punishing agents; (5) leads the individual to avoid contact with the environments where the punishment occurred, since these become conditioned aversive stimuli.

A fairly common example today is that of a teenager regarding *bullying*. Punishment from peers or the teacher in front of the school for poor performance (getting poor grades, asking questions considered "stupid", etc.) may (1) elicit responses incompatible with studying or test taking (e.g., tachycardia, tremor, dizziness, etc.— the famous "drawing a blank"); (2) establish the individual's own response as a source of aversive stimulation (studying, reading, testing, and asking questions in the classroom become aversive); (3) lead the individual to do any action that reduces the aversive stimulation caused by their own behavior (attacking peers or teachers, missing school, etc.); (4) lead the individual to avoid contact with punishing agents (social isolation both in the classroom and during breaks, such as in the case of students who spend their breaks in the library, in the bathroom, in the teachers' room, etc.); (5) lead the individual to avoid contact with the environments in which the punishments occurred (increase in the frequency of absences, absences from classrooms, or even withdrawal from school).

It should also be noted that typical MDD behaviors such as crying, complaining, expressing anxiety, and denial may be installed and maintained by positive reinforcement in the form of attention, care, love, help, companionship, etc. Even when reinforced, such behaviors are generally aversive to people who live with the depressed individual. In view of this, it is probable that they are affected by the passing of time, thus reducing the density of reinforcement obtained by the individual, which contributes to the permanence of the depressive condition (Dougher and Hackbert 1994; Kanter et al. 2005).

To date, the role of different forms of consequences on the installation and maintenance of the depressed behavior pattern was presented. Although this is a central factor in the behavior analytic understanding of the phenomenon, it is necessary to consider aspects related to discriminatory control, the individual's repertoire, and the verbal behavior.

As was pointed out, Lewinsohn and collaborators (1974) affirm that the unavailability of reinforcers due to environmental changes is a determining factor for depression (Lewinsohn 1974, 1975; Lewisohn and Libet 1972; Lewisohn et al. 1976). In this case, the environmental change refers to the loss of discriminative stimuli, or rather, of elements of the context that establish the occasion in which the response is usually being reinforced (Skinner 1965, 1991). An example of this is the death of the spouse, which implies not only the loss of important reinforcers but also the absence of the discriminative condition necessary for the production of reinforcement. It is fundamental to understand the difference between losing the reinforcer and losing the discriminative stimulus. In the first case, the individual gives the answer and the reinforcement does not happen. In the second case, the individual does not have the necessary environment for the emission of the response.

Another element that should be considered for the understanding of depression is whether the individual has the behavioral repertoire necessary to obtain certain types of reinforcers in different conditions. In particular, it is worth noting the inability to establish interpersonal relationships (i.e., social skills deficit; cf. Libet and Lewinsohn 1973) and to modify specific situations (problem-solving skills deficit; cf. Nezu 1986, 1987). Naturally, the lack of social and problem-solving skills repertoires can coexist with the other variables already discussed, as illustrated by Kanter et al. (2008): "a person who becomes depressed after a divorce, resulting in a reduction of the total positive reinforcement, and does not have adequate social skills to initiate new romantic relationships will probably become chronically depressed until the necessary social skills are learned" (Kanter et al. 2008, p. 5). Despite the relevance of the lack of social and problem-solving skills, it is worth noting that the absence of other behavioral repertoires may also favor a depressive condition. For example, in a study of 450 children in the fourth series, Cole (1990) found a strong correlation between academic difficulties and depression (Cole 1990).

Finally, it is important to examine the role that verbal behavior can play in the origin and permanence of a depressive situation. Kanter et al. (2005) explain that both the excess and the deficit of behaviors governed by rules are relevant to the understanding of the phenomenon (Kanter et al. 2005). The deficit in rules-governed behavior can make self-control difficult (i.e., the choice of immediate consequences and of lesser reinforcing value to the detriment of more distant consequences and of greater reinforcing value) and the capacity to solve problems. In turn, excessive behavior governed by rules may produce some degree of insensitivity to changes in contingencies and, therefore, be responsible for a rigidity of the repertoire that contributes to the clinical condition.

Yet as far as verbal behavior is concerned, some authors (e.g., Kanter et al. 2008; Törneke 2010), based on the paradigm of stimulus equivalence (Sidman 1994, 2000) and relational frame theory (RFT), *relational frame theory* (cf. Dymond and Roche 2013; Hayes et al. 2001; Perez et al. 2013) suggest that language considerably expands the range of situations that can contribute to the installation and maintenance of a depressive condition through the phenomenon of transference and the transformation of stimulus functions.

These authors understand language as the ability to create symbols by establishing arbitrary relationships between stimuli determined by the conviction of a verbal community. Human beings, in many contexts, are affected by symbols (written and spoken words, numbers, gestures, images, etc.) as they would be affected by the things to which these symbols refer (traditionally called referents; cf. De Rose and Bortoloti 2007). This is the phenomenon that has been studied in the research of stimulus equivalence and called transference of function.

Many experiments in stimulus equivalence have shown that, when a given stimulus belonging to a class of equivalent stimuli acquires a certain behavioral function (discriminative, elicitive, positive reinforcing, negative reinforcing), other stimuli belonging to that class indirectly acquire the same function (e.g., De Rose et al. 1988; for a review, see Dymond and Rehfeldt 2000).

As mentioned above, depressed patterns can have an escape and avoidance of aversive stimulation function, since the stimulus can begin to have an aversive elic-itive function (e.g., Hayes et al. 1991) or a negative reinforcement consequential function, since they are arbitrarily equivalent to other stimuli (that acquired these functions by direct contact with contingencies), the range of events that can acquire such functions expand considerably through symbolic action, contributing to the installation and maintenance of depressed patterns.

Therefore, a person who has learned, for example, that "giving up activities" is equivalent to "being problematic" or "having a mental problem" can avoid starting activities not because they have directly acquired an aversive function, but because giving up acquired an aversive function through the transfer of function. Thus, a pattern of avoiding the beginning of new activities can, in this case, diminish the production of positive reinforcers, installing and/or intensifying depressive conditions.

The expansion of the range of events that can acquire an aggressive function via function transference is even greater when it is considered that, in addition to creating symbols and reacting to them as if they were the lived or observed reality, we create symbols that refer only to other symbols and go on to react, also, to hypothesized realities:

> Similarly, the *origin of life*, *afterlife*, *the birth of the universe*, the events that no living person has ever experienced are therefore purely verbal constructions - words that are defined by other words. But then, having invented these words, we continue to build scientific and religious systems around them. Words become equivalent not only to observed reality, but also to hypothesized reality (Sidman 1994, p. 7).

An individual, when imagining "their own death", "their wake", thinking that there is no "life after death", these purely verbal constructions, may begin to feel elicited aversive stimuli and avoid the export of various situations equivalent to "run for your life". They can, in the extreme, do not leave the house, go to work, meet friends, etc. In this way, verbally constructed answers that in the short term produce avoidance of aversive stimulation, in the medium term will produce low density of positive reinforcement. Low tendency to agitation and feelings of unhappiness, sadness, and dissatisfaction are the expected products of this story.

In the late 1980s, experiments in the RFT area began to investigate other types of arbitrary relationships between stimuli, broadening the scope of analysis of phenomena related to cognition and language (Hayes et al. 2001). To the extent that the relationships established between the stimuli are not of equality, but of opposition, difference, comparison, hierarchy, among others, the function presented by arbitrarily related stimuli is not merely shared or transferred but transformed. In this way, a stimulus in opposition relationship with a positive reinforcer, for example, indirectly acquires the function of a negative reinforcer (Whelan and Barnes-Holmes 2004).

Experimental data on the transformation of stimulus function give Behavior Analysis even more explanatory power on complex human behavior, in general, and on the construction of depressed patterns, in particular, insofar as events of the world can acquire an aversive function if they are arbitrarily related as "opposed to" positively reinforcing events.

Some RFT research has shown that the verbal action of arbitrarily relating stimuli can produce the constitution of new aversive stimuli, at times even more powerful than those originally paired with unconditioned aversive stimuli. Dougher et al. (2007) investigated how arbitrary comparative relationships can affect the function of stimuli in a relational network (Dougher et al. 2007). In this research, three stimuli of similar dimensions (A, B, and C) were arbitrarily related in the following way: A as being the smallest, B as being the average, and C as the greatest (for descriptive purposes: A < B < C). It is worth highlighting that the stimuli were of the same size and, therefore, the comparative relationship between them was established arbitrarily and not in terms of the physical properties of these stimuli. After such arbitrary relationships were established, the B stimulus was paired with a shock. After successive pairings, the authors measured the magnitude of the elicited respondents (galvanic skin conductance) in relation to the stimuli A, B, and C and found that this varied according to the arbitrary relationship established. Thus, stimulus C, which had never been directly paired with the shock (aversive unconditioned stimulus), acquired a greater aversive value than stimulus B, which was directly paired with the aversive unconditioned stimulus. The authors concluded that the establishment of the arbitrary relationship "greater than" caused the participants to have a greater magnitude of elicited respondents in the presence of C (indirectly transformed aversive function) than in the presence of B (function acquired by direct contingencies of respondent conditioning). Anecdotal data indicate that such stimulus also acquired an aversive stimulus function by controlling the elusive operant: when C appeared, some participants removed the electrodes from the arm.

Whelan et al. (2006) demonstrated experimentally that stimuli can have their consequential functions transformed by means of arbitrary relations of comparison "more than" and "less than" (Whelan et al. 2006). In this experiment, a stimulus (D) acquired a positive reinforcing function by direct contingencies (its choice was occasioned by the three points gain). Stimuli E, F, and G were arbitrarily related as "more than" D, resulting, in descriptive terms, in the relationships D < E < F < G. Stimuli A, B, and C were arbitrarily listed as "less than" D, resulting in the following relationships A < B < C < D. The tests demonstrated that the consequential value of the stimuli that were arbitrarily related to D varied according to their participation in relational networks: G acquired a greater reinforcer value than F, F a greater value than E, and so on. Studies like this one seem to be of special importance to understand how the variation in the value of consequential events can, in humans, be a function of the relational response and not of the variations in the deprivation or intensity of the aversive stimulation. Since the prevalence of control by aversive stimulation and the low density of positive reinforcers are critical factors in depressive conditions, the understanding of how the relational response can be responsible for the acquisition and modulation of aversive and positive reinforcer consequential functions seems to be critical.

It is possible, for example, that a person who is watching the carnival parades on television, singing the music and feeling happy, may remember a time in which there was a carnival on the street and in which there was a comparison that it was "happier" at that time than now. This comparison can transform the positive reinforcing value of the present stimuli, in the sense of diminishing it. The person may stop singing, disconnect from the television, go to sleep, and refer to a feeling of sadness and melancholy. In another example, a student can have their grade thrown out on a test and feel very happy until they ask the teacher if they have a higher grade than the one given. Hearing that a student has earned an A, the previously reinforcing grade B may considerably lose its value, and the feeling of joy can be replaced by sadness and inferiority. Someone may think about the finitude of life and conclude that there is no life after death, speculate about the meaning of existence, and say that after this they feel completely unhappy, empty, and stop engaging in activities that have a given reinforcing value. This would also be an example of how the excess of control by verbal behavior can abolish positive reinforcing functions and contribute to the constituting of depressive patterns.

In short, verbal behavior, more specifically the arbitrarily applicable relational response, has an effect of transforming the environment, so that, depending on the idiosyncratic history of verbal learning, stimuli that could control a certain behavior may not do so, and other stimuli that supposedly do not control it may not do so. It is important to observe that both direct and indirect contingencies (i.e., established by means of verbal relationships) influence the individual's behavior pattern; therefore, the analysis of both is extremely relevant to the understanding of a case of depression.

Here, some interpretations for depression based on the experimental study of basic behavioral processes were presented. According to Donahoe (1993), the interpretation is a powerful tool for the understanding of diverse human behavioral phenomena, especially in cases that are too complex to be controlled experimentally or when the manipulation of variables would be unethical (Donahoe 1993). In addition to interpretation, another way of producing knowledge that is very relevant for the understanding of depression is with respect to experimental models of psychopathology.

The experimental models of psychopathology aim to produce, in controlled laboratory conditions, one or more characteristics of a given psychiatric disorder (Silva 2003). Although there are more than 18 experimental models of depression involving different animals (cf. Cryan and Slattery 2007; Willner 1984; Yan et al. 2010), this text presents only those that are more relevant to the present discussion, namely: chronic mild stress, learned helplessness, separation, and social defeat.

Or chronic mild stress (CMS) is an experimental model of depression in which they are exposed to various low-intensity stressors for an extended period of time. The protocol includes intermittent noise, inclination of the cage, alterations of the light-dark cycle, water and food deprivation, foul odor, presence of foreign objects, insertion of another animal in the cage, among others. Each one of the stressors is presented individually for some hours over approximately 6 weeks. Such exposure induces anhedonia (decrease in the capacity to feel pleasure), as measured by the significant reduction in the consumption of saccharine, which can persist for up to eight weeks (Willner 2005). In addition to anhedonia, the central symptom of depression, CMS produces a wide variety of symptoms present in a depressive condition, such as a decrease in locomotive activity (Gorka et al. 1996), weight loss (Willner et al. 1996), alterations in sound (Cheeta et al. 1997) and, still, it makes it difficult to establish discrimination (Rocha 2013).

The learned helplessness is a model of depression that evaluates the effects of the individual's contact with uncontrollable aggressive events. The experimental delineation consists of the separation of the subjects into three groups. In the first phase of the experiment, the subjects of Group 1 receive periodic shocks, which can be interrupted by the emission of a specific response previously determined by the researcher. The subjects of Group 2 are subjected to the same distribution of shocks with the same intensity and duration as the subjects of Group 1, but nothing they do can eliminate them, a condition defined as uncontrollability. Thus, when Group 1 subjects receive a shock, Group 2 subjects also receive a shock; when Group 1 subjects interrupt the shock, Group 2 subjects also stop the shock at the same time. Therefore, for the Group 2 subjects, the shock disappears independently of their actions, or in other words, there is no control relationship between their response and the withdrawal of the aversive stimuli. For their part, the Group 3 subjects do not undergo any experimental conditions. In the second phase of the experiment, all the subjects of all the groups are exposed to a new condition in which a new response (different from that which eliminates the shock in the previous phase) produces the elimination of shocks periodically presented in the experimental environment. In this second phase, then, all the subjects of all the groups could turn off the shock if they emitted the response previously specified by the researcher. In general, both Group 1 and Group 3 subjects learn the necessary response to eliminate the shock, but this does not occur with Group 2 subjects. Apparently, Group 2 subjects learn that there is no direct relationship between their actions and environmental changes, that is, they learn that their environment is uncontrollable (Hunziker 2005). In the case of human beings, the result of an experience of learned helplessness usually is a behavioral passivity associated with the notion that "nothing that I do make a difference," which is very common in depression (Overmie and LoLordo 1998).

Another experimental model of depression that deserves to be highlighted, even though it has been less studied than CMS and the lack of learning, is the separation model. In separation studies (e.g., Harlow and Suomi 1971, 1974; Hinde et al. 1978; Kaufman and Rosenblum 1967; Suomi et al. 1976), monkeys are isolated from their mothers and adult monkeys from their social environment for approximately 30 days, and all the basic conditions for survival (feeding, sound, etc.) are kept constant. Initially, the animals react to separation with agitation and screaming and, soon after, there is an overall decrease in all their behavior ("apathy"). When they are released for cohabitation with other monkeys, the subjects present a significant decrease in the locomotive activity, in the exploration of the environment, and in the search for interaction with other monkeys, in addition to arched physical posture, expressions of sadness and, in some cases, destructive behaviors. According to Hunziker (2006),

> the separation model mimics a type of human depression resulting from the deprivation of social reinforcers such as, for example, in cases of imprisonment, where the subject is totally removed from its reinforcer, or in cases of death/separation of a loved one, where the subject is deprived of the reinforcers for lack of the person who was their main source of reinforcement (Hunziker 2006, pp. 150–151).

In the social defeat model, a rat is introduced in the environment of another rat, larger and of a strain with a higher level of aggression. The "invader" rat is quickly attacked and defeated by the "resident" rat. After a few minutes of physical interaction, the two animals are separated by a transparent plastic partition with small holes, which allows visual, olfactory, and auditory contact between them, remaining in that condition for the next 24 hours. The experimental subject (smaller "invader" rat) is exposed to different "resident" rats every day for 1 or more weeks. This procedure produces a set of physiological and behavioral changes typical of depression, such as anhedonia, decrease in locomotive activity, exploratory behavior, and copulation initiative, among others (Huhman 2006). It is curious to note that collectively housed animals present reduced symptoms in comparison with animals housed alone, and that animals that live in more stable groups (with consolidated hierarchies and less intragroup aggression) present reduced symptoms in comparison with animals housed in an unstable group (De Jong et al. 2005).

In the following, the interpretative and experimental models previously presented will be used as an analytical tool for the understanding of how the cultural aspects of postmodernity are related to depression.

References

Biglan, A. (1991). Distressed behavior and its context. *The Behavior Analyst, 13*, 157–169.

Catania, A. C. (1999). *Learning: Behaviour, language and cognition* (4th ed.) (Souza, D. G. Trad.). Porto Alegre, RS: Artmed.

Cheeta, S., Ruigt, G., Van Proosdij, J., & Willner, P. (1997). Changes in sleep architecture following chronic mild stress. *Biological Psychiatry, 41*, 419–427.

Cole, D. A. (1990). The relation of social and academic competence to depressive symptoms in childhood. *Journal of Abnormal Psychology, 99*, 422–429.

Cryan, J. F., & Slattery, D. A. (2007). Animal models of mood disorders: Recent developments. *Current Opinion in Psychiatry, 20*, 1–7.

De Jong, J. G., Van der Vegt, B. J., Buwalda, B., & Koolhaas, J. M. (2005). Social environment determines the long-term effects of social defeat. *Physiology & Behavior, 84*, 87–95.

De Rose, J. C., & Bortoloti, R. (2007). The equivalence of stimuli as a model of meaning. *Acta Comportamentalia, 15*, 83–102.

De Rose, J. C., McIlvane, W. J., Dube, W. V., Galpin, V. C., & Stoddard, L. T. (1988). Emergent simple discrimination established by indirect relation to differential consequences. *Journal of the Experimental Analysis of Behavior, 50*, 1–20.

Donahoe, J. W. (1993). The unconventional wisdom of B. F. Skinner: The analysis-interpretation distinction. *Journal of the Experimental Analysis of Behavior, 60*, 453–456.

Dougher, M. J., & Hackbert, L. (1994). A behavior-analytic account of depression and a case report using acceptance-based procedures. *The Behavior Analyst, 17*, 321–334.

Dougher, M., Hamilton, D., Brandi, C., Fink, C., & Harrington, J. (2007). Transformation of the discriminative and eliciting functions of generalized relational stimuli. *Journal of the Experimental Analysis of Behavior, 88*, 179–187.

Dymond, S., & Rehfeldt, R. A. (2000). Understanding complex behavior: The transformation of stimulus functions. *The Behavior Analyst, 23*, 239–254.

Dymond, S., & Roche, B. (2013). *Advances in relational frame theory: Research and application.* Oakland: New Harbinger.

Ferster, C. B. (1973). A functional analysis of depression. *American Psychologist, 28*, 857–870.

Ferster, C. B., & Skinner, B. F. (1957). *Schedules of reinforcement.* New York, NY: Appleton-Century-Crofts.

Gorka, Z., Moryl, E., & Papp, M. (1996). Effect of chronic mild stress on circadian rhythms in the locomotor activity in rats. *Pharmacology Biochemistry and Behavior, 54*, 229–234.

Harlow, H. F., & Suomi, S. J. (1971). Production of depressive behavior in young monkeys. *Journal of Autism and Childhood Schizophrenia, 1*, 246–255.

Harlow, H. F., & Suomi, S. J. (1974). Induced depression in monkeys. *Behavioral Biology, 12*, 273–296.

Hayes, S. C., Barnes-Holmes, D., & Roche, B. (Eds.). (2001). *Relational frame theory: A post-Skinnerian account of human language and cognition.* New York, NY: Plenum Press.

Hayes, S. C., Kohlenberg, B. S., & Hayes, L. J. (1991). The transfer of specific and general consequential functions through simple and conditional equivalence relations. *Journal of the Experimental Analysis of Behavior, 56*, 119–137.

Hinde, R. A., Leighton-Shapiro, M. E., & McGinnis, L. (1978). Effects of various types of separation experience on rhesus monkeys 5 months later. *Journal of Child Psychology and Psychiatry, 19*, 199–211.

Huhman, K. L. (2006). Social conflict models: Can they inform us about human psychopathology? *Hormones and Behavior, 50*, 640–646.

Hunziker, M. H. L. (2005). Or learned helplessness revisited: Estudos com animais. *Psychology: Theory and Research, 21*, 131–139.

Hunziker, M. H. L. (2006). Estudo experimental da depressão. In H. J. Guilhardi & N. C. Aguirre (Eds.), *On behavior and cognition* (Vol. 18, pp. 149–155). Santo André, SP: ESETec.

Kanter, J. W., Busch, A. M., Weeks, C. E., & Landes, S. J. (2008). The nature of clinical depression: Symptoms, syndromes, and behavior analysis. *The Behavior Analyst, 31*, 1–21.

Kanter, J. W., Callaghan, G. M., Landes, S. J., Busch, A. M., & Brown, K. R. (2004). Behavior analytic conceptualization and treatment of depression: Traditional models and recent advances. *The Behavior Analyst Today, 5*, 255–274.

Kanter, J. W., Cautilli, J. D., Busch, A. M., & Baruch, D. E. (2005). Toward a comprehensive functional analysis of depressive behavior: Five environmental factors and a possible sixth and seventh. *The Behavior Analyst Today, 6*, 65–81.

Kanter, J. W., Landes, S. J., Busch, A. M., Rusch, L. C, Baruch, D. E., & Manos, R. C. (2007). An integrative model of depression using modern behavioral principles. In D. W. Woods & J. W. Kanter (Eds.), *Understanding behavior disorders: A contemporary behavioral perspective* (pp. 181–215). Reno: Context Press.

Kaufman, I. C., & Rosenblum, L. A. (1967). The reaction to separation in infant monkeys: Anaclitic depression and conservation-withdrawal. *Psychosomatic Medicine, 29*, 648–675.

Lewinsohn, P. M. (1974). A behavioral approach to the treatment of depression. In R. M. Freidman & M. M. Katz (Eds.), *The psychology of depression: Contemporary theory and research* (pp. 157–185). New York, NY: Wiley.

Lewinsohn, P. M. (1975). The behavioral study and treatment of depression. In M, Hersen, R. M. Eisler, & P. M. Miller (Eds.), *Progress in behavior modification* (pp. 19–64). New York, NY: Academic Press.

Lewisohn, Biglan, A., & Zeiss, A. S. (1976). Behavioral treatment of depression. In P. O. Davidson (Ed.), *The behavioral management of anxiety, depression and pain* (pp. 91–146). New York, NY: Brunner/Mazel.

Lewisohn, P. M., & Libet, J. (1972). Pleasant events, activity schedules and depression. *Journal of Abnormal Psychology, 79*, 291–295.

Libet, J. M., & Lewinsohn, P. M. (1973). The concept of social skill with special reference to the behavior of depressed persons. *Journal of Consulting and Clinical Psychology, 40*, 304–312.

Nezu, A. M. (1986). Efficacy of a social problem-solving therapy approach for unipolar depression. *Journal of Consulting and Clinical Psychology, 54*, 196–202.

Nezu, A. M. (1987). A problem-solving formulation of depression: A literature review and proposal of a pluralistic model. *Clinical Psychology Review, 7*, 121–144.

Overmier, J. B., & LoLordo, V. M. (1998). Learned helplessness. In W. O'Donohue (Ed.), *Learning and behavior therapy* (pp. 352–373). Boston: Allyn and Bacon.

Perez, W. F., Nico, Y. C., Kovac, R., Fidalgo, A. P., & Leonardi, J. L. (2013). Introduction to relational frame theory: Main concepts, experimental studies and application possibilities. *Perspectives in Behavior Analysis, 4*(1), 33–51.

Rocha, L. M. (2013). *The effects of chronic mild stress on the establishment of discrimination.* (Dissertação de mestrado), Pontifícia Universidade Católica de São Paulo, São Paulo, SP.

Sidman, M. (1994). *Equivalence relations and behavior: A research story.* Boston: Authors Cooperative.

Sidman, M. (2000). Equivalence relations and the reinforcement contingency. *Journal of the Experimental Analysis of Behavior, 74*, 127–146.

Silva, M. T A. (2003). *Behavioural models in neurosciences* (Tese de livre docência). São Paulo, SP: University of São Paulo.

Skinner, B. F. (1965). *Science and human behavior.* New York, NY: Free Press (Original work published in 1953).

Skinner, B. F. (1976). *About behaviorism.* New York, NY: Vintage Books (Original work published in 1974).

Skinner, B. F. (1991). *The behavior of organisms: An experimental analysis.* Acton: Copley (Original work published in 1938).

Suomi, S. J., Collins, M. L., & Harlow, H. F. (1976). Effect of maternal and peer separations on young monkeys. *Journal of Child Psychology and Psychiatry, 17*, 101–112.

Törneke, N. (2010). *Learning RFT: An introduction to relational frame theory and its clinical application.* Reno: Context Press.

Whelan, R., & Barnes-Holmes, D. (2004). The transformation of consequential functions in accordance with the relational frames of same and opposite. *Journal of the Experimental Analysis of Behavior, 82*, 177–195.

Whelan, R., Barnes-Holmes, D., & Dymond, S. (2006). The transformation of consequential functions in accordance with the relational frames of more-than and less-than. *Journal of the Experimental Analysis of Behavior, 86*, 317–335.

Willner, P. (1984). The validity of animal models of depression. *Psychopharmacology, 83*, 1–16.

Willner, P. (2005). Chronic mild stress (CMS) revisited: Consistency and behavioural-neurobiological concordance in the effects of CMS. *Neuropsychobiology, 52*, 90–110.

Willner, P., Moreau, J. L., Nielsen, C. K., Papp, M., & Sluzewska, A. (1996). Decreased hedonic responsiveness following chronic mild stress is not secondary to loss of body weight. *Physiology & Behavior, 60*, 129–134.

Yan, H. C., Cao, X., Das, M., Zhu, X. H, & Gao, T. M. (2010). Behavioral animal models of depression. *Neuroscience Bulletin, 26*, 327–337.

Chapter 3
Depression and Culture: A Diagnosis of Our Time

The contemporary era is called postmodern and may be considered a period of economic and social transformations observed since the last quarter of the twentieth century. To understand it, it is necessary to trace the historical course of the development of western civilization since premodernity. In this view, a brief characterization of pre-modern societies will be presented, with the objective of highlighting, later, how modern societies established a new beginning of social contingencies and, with that, the basis for the emergence of a new notion of individual. In this second moment, some factors related to the production of depression as a cultural phenomenon will be highlighted (Ferreira and Tourinho 2011). Having made this journey, the economic and social transformations identified in the last quarter of the twentieth century will be exposed, inaugurating a new era of capitalism, and marking the passage from modern society to the postmodern. In this last moment, the defining characteristics of postmodernity will be presented with a view of providing elements that help think about the possible ways in which the new social uprooting can contribute to the promotion of depression in the lives of human beings today. Therefore, analyses will be explored by philosophers, social scientists, psychiatrists, and psychologists on the main changes that constitute postmodernity. These analyses will serve as material to analyze the social determinants of depression in the present. The interpretative and experimental models of depression existing in Behavior Analysis will be used as an analytical tool.

3.1 Premodern and Modern Societies

In premodern societies, the survival of each individual was in every way related to the survival of others. The organization of social life occurred in terms of collective needs. Thus, the objectives of the individual and the group were, for the most part, coincidental. Once external threats were the dominant trend, the survival of each

Y. Nico et al., *Depression as a Cultural Phenomenon in Postmodern Society*, SpringerBriefs in Psychology, https://doi.org/10.1007/978-3-030-60545-2_3

individual was more probable if there was mutual cooperation. Therefore, the group members acted and thought from the point of view of "we" and not of "me" (Elias 1990, 1994).

In feudal societies, more specifically, professional, social, and private lives were not dissociated. It is clear that the houses do not have defined spaces for each function. There was no place for secrets, intimacy, or privacy—all these were social constructions of later periods (Ariés 1981). In this way, these societies were not individualized and there were no aspects of life that were private.

The communities lived in fiefdoms and the Church, with its Christian paternalistic ethic, recommended that the property owners should protect others without material interests or gains. In feudal life, social mobility was practically nonexistent and individual functions were predefined according to the social group of birth. In this society, nobles and servants had different rights and duties, and changes in social status were rare (Ariés and Duby 1990). Therefore, plans for individual conquests did not constitute an object of personal reflection, and it was necessary to evaluate other alternatives for life projects (Elias 1990, 1994; Tourinho 2009). Eventually, reflections on other aspects of life, when realized, occurred publicly (Ariés 1981; Ariés and Duby 1990; Sennett 1988). It is clear that, in feudal societies, individuals do not need social valuation to obtain individual interests and do not need to plan long-term goals.

Another defining aspect of feudal sociability refers to the absence of a notion of childhood; of an idea that children were substantially different from adults; and of specific feelings related to childhood. The children were pampered only when they were very young, like pets and later, they were already considered a man or a young woman. They lived mixed with adults and learned their daily tasks, doing with adults what they did. Affective exchanges and social communications also took place outside the family, in a "dense and intimate" collective environment (Ariés 1981).

Another factor that deserves to be highlighted is the relationship of the feudal individual with time. According to Ricouer (1975), time control is the oldest and most permanent form of social control, since, in different cultures, individuals have never been able to organize their daily time in a way that is totally independent of the group (Ricouer 1975). In premodern agrarian civilizations, the temporal experience was very much regulated by the cycles of nature: moments of planting and harvesting; daytime moments for work; nighttime moments for rest, etc. The firsthand clocks, without seconds, placed on church towers date from the end of the Middle Ages. Nature's time was thus punctuated by religious time. The ringing of the church bell signaled the hour of awakening, the birth of someone, the hour of the Hail Mary, etc. (Ricouer 1975).

Transformations in agricultural technologies and in the means of transportation, in addition to the increase of productivity with surpluses and the population and urban growth, mark the end of the Middle Ages, between the XI and XIII centuries. The monetarization of economic functions and productive activities led to the appearance of the first suburbs and of a new social class—the bourgeoisie—made up of merchants.

The new material conditions of existence, founded by the growing search for profit and the strengthening of market relations, developed in connection with new forms of religion. Luther's Protestant Reformation is an example of a new ethic that ideologically supported the accumulation of capital, exalting the materialistic motivations, greed, profit, and selfishness, once condemned in feudalism (Tourinho 2009). Thus, we are witnessing the gradual destruction of the social foundations of feudalism and the emergence of the modern era.

The modern era refers to the period of consolidation of the capitalist mode of production in the place of the feudal mode of production, with the Industrial Revolution in the eighteenth century being a defining framework of its beginning. The following will briefly describe the central transformations in this period.

Burgs grew and gave rise to the appearance and complexity of the first cities. Thus, the administrative time to organize urban life arises. Clocks began to exist not only in the towers of the churches but also in the towers of city hall, indicating the emergence of another group, in addition to the religious one, with the power to control the life of individuals (Ricouer 1975). The process of strengthening this administrative-political power culminated in the formation of unified national states, with Portugal being the first nation-state to appear in the fourteenth century and Italy and Germany the last in the nineteenth century.

Given the new economic bases, social mobility became possible, being dependent on individual empowerment. The social functions were no longer defined by birth, and several possible courses of action were placed in the individual horizon. The increasing expansion of the possibilities of choices was accompanied by a greater quantity of passive opportunities to be "lost." The future of the individual became, clearly, more uncertain and a subject of pressure (Tourinho 2009).

The State, as an impersonal power, began to regulate economic relations, to provide conditions for individuals to separate themselves from their groups of origin and to assume the function of protecting and mediating social relations (Elias 1990, 1994). The loss of security provided by the original reference group and the increase of the degree of individualization and solidarity configure the period that Bruckner (1996) called *the age of eternal torment.*

While in the Middle Ages the forms of everyday life were not very varied, being regulated by the Church. During the Renaissance, a period of transition from feudalism to the modern age, social relations became the subject of a literature of civility that postulated codes of etiquette and conduct. This "civilizing process" was marked by fundamental alterations in the relationships of individuals between themselves and with their own bodies, promoting a modesty that did not exist until that point in relation to the parts and functions of the body, strict emotional control and self-control, instead of spontaneity in relationships (Elias 1990, 1994).

According to Elias (1990, 1994), the maintenance of civility, with its coordinated, foreseeable standards and control of individual behavior, became fundamental for the functioning of a new social order characterized by more extensive commercial relations and increasingly differentiated social functions. These new social demands required that individuals perform a careful self-observation of bodily functions, emotional states, thoughts, and emotions so that, in this way, they can control unwanted social actions. The importance of distinguishing between what should be reserved for the intimate life and, in the last instance, be felt and thought "within itself" and what could be expressed for the other led to the constituting of the "invisible wall of emotions" (Elias 1990, 1994).

Exactly because the complex social networks with indirect relationships obscure the interdependence that exists between the functions performed by very distant members, individuals in modern societies have come to think and feel as autonomous and separate from others, as if they were encapsulated in themselves, as *homoclausus* (Elias 1990, 1994). Then emerges the concept of an "inner self," "intimate," taken as "true self" and totally apart from those who are in the outside world—the society.

Therefore, according to Elias (1990, 1994), the greater degree of interdependence between individuals in modern Western societies was accompanied by the promotion and refinement of individual self-control, the appearance of a concept of interiority of feelings and thoughts, and a greater restriction on impulsiveness[1] (Elias 1990, 1994).

The perception of time has also brought about a profound transformation in modern times. The daily time passed to be marked by the production. The consolidation of the capitalist mode of production, which defined modern societies, took place with the Industrial Revolution in the eighteenth century, and it was at this time that the recluses began to appear in the factories, establishing the time of production that we live with today. In capitalism, for the first time in history, part of the time is expropriated from the worker, constituting the most important value (Kehl 2009). "Modern times," eternalized by Chaplin's work, are times of acceleration for the accumulation of capital. "Time is money" had already become a commonplace statement.

Finally, it is worth noting that, concomitant with the process of transition from feudalism to capitalism, the social invention of childhood was given. The children, who in premodern life grew up together with adults learning in daily life to perform various daily activities, were separated to be socialized in school, an institution created in the eighteenth century. This enclosure—schooling—became necessary not only to transmit the innumerable knowledge required in adult life but also to "domesticate" impulses and to teach self-controlled patterns (Ariés 1981).

Such a process would not have been possible without sentimental complicity of the families. The family became a necessary place of affection between the couple and between parents and children, which did not happen in feudal society. The appearance of the socializing function of the family also dates from the eighteenth century. The family, as a new social institution, began to organize itself around the child, its main role being to ensure and control their socialization (Ariés 1981).

In this new context, the house acquired a new function: it changed the place where the family gathered in collective spaces and exerted affectivity. The street, the square, and public spaces were no longer the place where the "dense and warm" exchanges occurred. They happened to occur with the family and around the child, evidencing the disappearance of the old sociability. The house became better prepared

---

[1]For a systematization of the thought of Norbert Elias, see Tourinho (2009).

for intimacy, in which the functional independence of comfort and communication through the corridor arises.

This period of preparation for adult life, which began with the advent of childhood, was gradually extended to the emergence of adolescence, another social construction, in the nineteenth century. As the social functions of the capitalist-industrial society became more complex and specialized, the waiting period for entering adult life was also expanded. Individuals, even though they were no longer children and presented sexual safety for reproduction, were no longer incorporated into adult life, and were not considered suitable for marriage. However, they had already acquired the physical capacities of the adult—strength, dexterity, ability, coordination, etc. They were then considered too immature, intellectually and emotionally, to enter the labor market. This period of moratorium seems to be of fundamental importance to understand the values of contemporary culture and its relationship with the production of depression in the present day (Kehl 2004), which will be further discussed in the analysis of depression produced in postmodernity.

The interpretative analyses offered in this book about possible cultural determinants of depression in postmodern societies are organized around the thematic axes that structured the historical narrative up to this point in the text, namely: the patterns of sociability; the relations of the subject with its own body; the daily temporal experience and the social constructions in relation to adolescence. Before continuing with the considerations on how these aspects appear in the life of the postmodern human being, it is worth presenting an behavior analytic interpretation, elaborated by Ferreira and Tourinho (2011), on depression in modern societies.

3.2 Modernity and Depression

The establishment of the capitalist mode of production occurred after a long period of social, political, economic, and cultural transformations. Among the changes that accompanied the consolidation of modern capitalist societies was the emergence of a new way of seeing, feeling, and thinking about oneself. The advent of a modern western conception of the individual as an autonomous individual, independent of others, is a central aspect of these individualized societies. Given the new conception, the problems considered as subjective were also delineated and treated in a new way. Depression, as a cultural phenomenon, was configured in a particular way in modern individualized societies (Ferreira and Tourinho 2011; Tourinho 2009).

Ferreira and Tourinho (2011), for example, list central aspects that constitute depression and assume several cultural variables related to the phenomenon (Ferreira and Tourinho 2011). The sensations of "apprehension about the future" and of "incompetence and failure" may be related to the way in which childhood and adolescence are lived in modern times. Considering that, in these phases, individuals do not exercise many of the activities demanded in adult life (many times, even being exposed to the outbursts of contingencies that are incomparable with those typical of the adult period), a feeling of "pressure regarding the future" and of "incompetence and failure" to deal with new future contingencies seems to be a predictable collateral product. Perhaps, for this reason, it is observed that adolescence is a critical period for the initiation of psychopathological symptoms (Kehl 2004).

Another cultural factor that presumably produces a constant feeling of "incompetence and failure" is the organized contingencies in an individualized society. Individuals are required to make their own decisions and choices independently and are offered, in the modern industrialized world, an increasingly wide range of consumption possibilities and life courses. They must deal with the "weight" of the renunciations made, of the possibilities lost, of the lives not lived. This is particularly acute in a society that attributes to the individual, seen as independent of others, the responsibility for their own success or failure. A world with new aversive conditioned stimulus then comes to exist, thus, establishing new conditions for the strengthening of escape and avoidance patterns of possible social failures.

It is easy to imagine, therefore, that feelings of "incompetence and failure" are produced by these social contingencies, and that depressed patterns may assume an escape and avoidance function of these types of social disapproval. Add to this fact that, in those societies, specific cultural contingencies spread

> Several well-succeeded professional models, lifestyles based on unrestrained consumption and a permanent good life as a result of the rules - the value of contingencies is increased, in which there is no positive reinforcement with respect to a certain activity, as long as an ideal model is under control (Ferreira and Tourinho 2011, p. 30).

Thus, verbal reports about "incompetence or failure" become more possible in societies, such as individualized ones, which deal with contingencies in this way.

Another important analysis presented by Ferreira and Tourinho (2011) refers to the self-descriptive standards produced in modern societies and their control over the behavior of individuals (Ferreira and Tourinho 2011). Since the concept of the individual, in modernity, is that of a being whose nature was not built on a relationship with others, socially recriminated patterns of behavior can be considered as an expression of a nature or personality of the individual, generally conceived as immutable.

To the extent that these societies encourage demonstrations of autonomy and independence, it is common to observe the members of the social group releasing aggressive consequences when demonstrations of dependence and passivity are considered inadequate. Returning to the example from the beginning of this book, in which the person spends the whole day in bed and does not go to work with the intention of avoiding a meeting in which they would probably be reprimanded, it is possible to imagine that they may come into contact with reprimands from their spouse, as being called "fragile," "dependent," "disturbed" and acquires a self-destructive repertoire that goes on to control other behaviors. Such control can be especially strong and permanent if we consider that

> the self-image of the modern man based on an inner self isolated from the external world will strengthen the notion of feelings and emotions intrinsic to the nature of the individual, leaving aside the fact that they constitute established components in the relationship of individuals with others (Ferreira and Tourinho 2011, p. 31).

The relationship with death in modern Western societies is also analyzed by Ferreira and Tourinho (2011) as a possible aspect related to depression (Ferreira and Tourinho 2011). In premodern societies, the death of a group member was part of everyday life, it was lived with the same naturalness as other everyday facts and constituted a public event. In modern societies, the relationship with death is completely different: death is not left with tranquility and the subject is treated as a social taboo; the event is privatized and, many times, it does not occur in the family environment so that it is treated hygienically in specific locations; finally, the removal of death, effectively or as a possible occurrence, is the norm. The authors suggest that this modern western attitude toward death can make it difficult to acquire a more adaptive behavioral repertoire when the exposure to real contingencies involving the death of a loved one has repercussions on the way individuals experience a significant loss with a high reinforcing value, a factor associated with depression.

From the observation that existing practices in modern Western societies were producing sad, unsatisfied, and depressed individuals, Skinner (1986) asked a question that became the title of the article *Or what is Wrong with Everyday Life in the Western World?* The "diagnosis" from which it originates is stated at the very beginning of the text (Skinner 1986):

> Many of those who live in Western democracies enjoy a great deal of freedom, security and freedom. But they have their own problems. Despite their privileges, many are hated, restless or depressed. They are not enjoying their lives. They don't like what they do: they don't do what they like. In a word, they are unhappy. This is not the most serious problem in the world, but it can be said to be a definite problem (p. 568).

It should be noted that, from the outset, Skinner (1986) clearly outlines the problem he intends to discuss. It is a phenomenon relative to "Western democracies," a "problem of the world" or, as he also puts it further, a phenomenon produced by the "current lifestyle of the West" (Skinner 1986, p. 568). As a result of this demarcation, the author launches into the exercise of identifying and interpreting, based on the principles of Behavior Analysis, existing cultural practices in the "daily life of the Western world" that could respond to the question "what is wrong?" The term "wrong" makes special sense because Skinner starts from the recognition that the Western *way of life* is the one coveted by most of the world. Therefore, already from the beginning, Skinner indicates his starting point: the same cultural practices exalted for producing well-being and happiness are, in a not so obvious way, also producers of tedium, indifference, dissatisfaction, and depression.

In developing this analysis and facing the question of what would need to be changed for individuals to feel these cultures in other ways, Skinner (1986) makes a distinction between two effects of reinforcement: pleasure and strengthening.

> I would like to make a distinction between the effects of pleasure and strengthening. They occur at different times and are felt as different things. When we feel satisfied, we are not necessarily inclined to behave in the same way. On the other hand, when we repeat a behavior that was reinforced, we do not feel the same pleasant effect that we felt at the moment the reinforcement took place. Pleasure seems to be the word of the day that is closest to the reformer, but it only takes on the effect (Skinner 1986, p. 569).

From the analysis of these two effects, the author defends that the cultural practices of Western societies evolved, fundamentally, in the direction of promoting the pleasant effect of reinforcement, neglecting the strengthening effect. Thus, the contingencies provided by the modern Western culture have corroded certain relationships with the environment that result in the strengthening of behavior. Skinner (1986) analyzes five practices that are central to the constituting of this culture and that has promoted the loss of most of the strengthening effects of the behavior consequences at the expense of promoting pleasing effects (Skinner 1986). They are the alienation of the worker; welfarism; the widespread following of advice; the following of ethical and legal rules; the promotion of passive behaviors.

In analyzing worker alienation, Skinner (1986) argues that the process of industrialization involved a separation between work behavior and the type of immediate consequences that modeled and maintained the worker's behavior, i.e., the immediate and intrinsic consequences that were contingent upon work ceasing to exist (Skinner 1986). While in precapitalist societies, individuals gave different answers to the work (a craftsman, for example, made the shoe alone, treated the leather, built forms, placed the leather in these forms, sewed the leather on its own, etc., until the shoe was ready), in industrial societies, the work was specialized. The Industrial Revolution brought with it the beginning of the era of repetition of a single behavior in the world of work (see the criticism contained in the famous dinner of Chaplin's self-employed worker, who repeated, without any effort, the gesture of tightening a screw, even when it was not before them in the production line). Thus, the contingencies of reinforcement of behavioral variability were replaced by contingencies of reinforcement of behavioral stereotype.

As this arrangement of contingencies produces a tendency to weaken behavior, because even what one wants to do loses its intrinsic reinforcing value when exposed to repetition (e.g., Ariely et al. 2008), aversive contingencies are released by the employers to maintain the strength of the employees' behavior. As the immediate and intrinsic consequences of working are no longer reinforcing, the arbitrary consequence—*money*—is released to strengthen such behavior. Meanwhile, as in industrialized societies, most of the working population receives a payment for the amount of time worked (interval schemes) and not in schemes depending on the responses of working strictly on demand (payment per piece or commission), the supplementation of the control of the working behavior is made with aversive contingencies. Thus, the prevalence of aversive control is noted to the detriment of control by positive reinforcement of the contingent emission of responses—or of response chains—to work. Working to avoid losing one's job will inevitably be accompanied by feelings of dissatisfaction, discouragement, unhappiness, tedium, and little inclination to act, all of which are present in depression.

In addition, industrialization involved the gradual replacement of human work by mechanical work. More recently, in the history of capitalism, technological development has led to the construction of devices to support our efforts and increase the speed of execution of daily tasks, after all, "time is money". As Skinner (1986) points out:

Consider the extent to which the mechanisms that work for us have become button openers. We opened buttons in elevators, telephones, panels, videos, washing machines, furnaces, writing machines and computers, all in exchange for actions that had at least a little bit of variety (Skinner 1986, p. 570).

It is worth mentioning that the article *Or what is Wrong with Everyday Life in the Western World?* (Skinner 1986) dates back to the mid-1980s, and from then to now, technological development has brought about an acceleration never before seen, especially in the area of information technology and communication systems, which has placed modern capitalist society in a new phase, called postmodernity. As a result, the occupation of "button pressers" has become a daily occurrence, further restricting behavioral variability and accelerating the daily pace in an unprecedented way. These two aspects, which have their beginnings in modernity and are related to the production of depressed patterns, intensified in postmodernity, as it will be explained later.

The second practice analyzed is the welfarism which, by valuing the "doing for the other," often promotes actions of help when the other would have the conditions to do so by themself. Thus, it prevents the strengthening of autonomous and useful behaviors in the life of those who receive assistance and the opportunity to engage in pleasant activities. In their eagerness to spare individuals the effort to respond, from frustrations they have to face and problems they have to solve, it makes it impossible for them to be in contact with the consequences that strengthen behavior.

It is known, for example, that a greater value is attributed to a product when it is produced by the individual himself than when it is made by another person (e.g., Norton et al. 2012). Benevolent practices run the risk of strengthening more passive classes of behavior, such as asking for help, complaining of incompetence to do things, saying that one does not know how to do things, and depreciating oneself, to the detriment of more active classes of behavior. It is not surprising, that there is, as a result of this history, a deficit in repertoire to act associated with excessive verbalizations of complaints due to inabilities and feelings of lack of motivation and uselessness, aspects that are also described in the diagnosis of depression.

The strengthening effect of reinforcement is lost in a third way "when people do things just because they are given them to do." In Western cultures, there has been a great expansion of this behavior "governed by rules" (Skinner 1986). Although Skinner does not discuss why the control of behavior by rules has been especially widespread in those societies, it is possible to overcome it, based on the examples provided by him, because these societies are based on consumption. In his words: "they buy the car they were told to buy; they see the movie they were told to see; they buy it at the store they were told to buy it." The excessive governed by rules behaviors are yet another source of restricted variability. By avoiding the cost of exploring new contingencies, the type of strengthening effect that is generated by experienced consequences is lost.

The fourth practice analyzed by Skinner (1986) also refers to behavior governed by rules, but, in this case, the rules that are followed to please or avoid displeasing others, called "laws" (p. 571), while the rules that were described above are called "advice" (p. 570) (Skinner 1986). This type of control, which Skinner (1986) calls "control by ethical rules" (p. 571), promotes special corrosion of the strengthening effect when such rules are replaced by laws (Skinner 1986). This happens because the following laws are generally negatively reinforced—or rather, it happens primarily to avoid punishment—and because, in general, governmental and religious laws are kept for the benefit of institutions and, when they act on behalf of the individual, the strengthening consequences are indirect and very delayed. In addition, as cultural practices change more quickly than rules and laws, people generally "do what is right" for reasons that are no longer advantageous to anyone.

The last cultural practice analyzed by Skinner (1986) is the excessive reinforcement of "passive" behavior. Western cultures have become experts in providing immediate and pleasing consequences (Skinner 1986). Attractive, captivating, curious, funny, nice, and charming things are produced and collected as objects of fun, but they reinforce little else to be smelled, tasted, attended, read, and enjoyed.

> It may not seem that someone doesn't enjoy a life spent smelling good food, eating delicious meals, attending interesting performances and playing. But it would be a life in which nothing else would be done, and few of those who were able to tempt it were remarkably happy. What is wrong with life in the West is not that it has too many reinforcers, but that the reinforcers are not contingent on the types of behavior that support the individual or promote the survival of the culture or the species (Skinner 1986, p. 571).

In short, the cultural practices of the West produced a weakening of behavior by sacrificing the strengthening consequences for the promotion of merely pleasing consequences; by substituting natural reinforcers for arbitrary, conditioned and generalized reinforcers; by distending the temporal relationship between response and consequence (as in the case of the following of rules); and by promoting stereotypical behavior in the place of variability.

3.3   Postmodernity and Depression

From the last quarter of the twentieth century, the increase in the capitalist system of production led to profound economic, social, and political transformations. Exactly because the intensification and pervasiveness of typical characteristics of capitalist societies produced unprecedented impacts in different spheres of social and individual life, some authors distinguish this period by calling it postindustrial capitalism, multinational capitalism, postconsumer capitalism, poststructuralist capitalism, postmodernity, and liquid modernity (Bauman 2001). It seems, therefore, that the understanding of aspects of contemporary capitalist society, among them the high prevalence of depression diagnosis, requires a proper examination.

Skinner (1986) had already observed, in the middle of the 1980s (i.e., at the moment of the passage from modernity to postmodernity), that unhappiness, tedium, empathy, and dissatisfaction were products of cultural practices promoted by the desired Western lifestyle (Skinner 1986). In addition, it was not, according to him, a product of any kind. Skinner (1986) argued that these problems affect a large proportion of the individuals in these societies. It was, therefore, a phenomenon of western capitalist culture (Skinner 1986). If, at that moment in history, the prevailing social contingencies already seemed to be promoting depression, it is possible that the emergence of capitalism was accompanied by the intensification of the problematic aspects identified by Skinner and, perhaps, by the emergence of new social practices promoting depression. Is there anything more wrong with the daily life of the Western world today?

Data from epidemiological research seem to answer, "yes": the prevalence of MDD over the course of life is higher in developed countries than in developing ones (Kessler and Üstün 2008), and the lower prevalence of MDD was found in Japan which, although it is a developed country (and, therefore, with a globalized economy), still preserves cultural practices of the Eastern world. What is especially wrong with the life promoted in the postmodern societies of the West? Why do developed countries, in comparison with developing countries, have produced a greater number of individuals with depression over the course of their lives? In developing countries, the highest rate of depression was reached in São Paulo, Brazil (Kessler and Üstün 2008). Why? Whatever the answers are, it is very clear that they are not genetic. The factors responsible for the high prevalence of depression in the contemporary Western world, in general, and in developed countries in particular, are most likely of a social nature.

Another argument in favor of a cultural understanding of the phenomenon of depression is the tendency to increase the number of cases with this diagnosis—as noted above, MDD was classified in the GBD of 1990 as the fourth major cause of death, moving to the third in 2000 and second in 2010, with estimates of reaching first place in 2030 (Bromet et al. 2011; Lépine and Briley 2011). This suggests that the cultural practices promoting depression have had an exponential impact.

Many authors have set out to analyze possible relationships between contemporary cultural practices and the promotion of depression. Roughly speaking, the literature on the subject can be divided into two major research fronts, the principle of which is compatible with each other: one that seeks to identify social changes produced by current capitalism and their impact on the daily lives of individuals (e.g., Bauman 2001, 2004a, b, 2013; Ferreira and Tourinho 2011; Hidaka 2012; James 1998, 2007a, b, 2008; Kessler 1997; Kehl 2004, 2009; Lafrance 2009; Pickett and Wilkinson 2010) and another that discusses changes in the cultural practices of diagnosing and treating depression as an important variable for understanding the high prevalence of this diagnosis (e.g., Burns 2013; Geaney 2011; Pardo and Pérez-Álvarez 2007; Pessotti 2001).

The following text will prioritize the analyses on social changes that characterize postmodernity, since carefully exploring these two research fronts extrapolates the objectives of this book. In the final part of the text, some elements of the discussion on changes in the cultural practices of diagnosis and treatment of depression will be presented. This last topic certainly deserves to be the object of future research to provide a more complete picture of the relationship between culture and depression today.

The passage from modernity to postmodernity is identified, on the socioeconomic level, by the emergence and strengthening of multinationals, the intensification of the approximation of the financial markets of different countries, the narrowing of economic, social, political, and cultural interactions, constituting the so-called "global village" (McLuhan and Fiore 1969). The globalization of the economy has allowed developed countries to expand their consumer market beyond the internal market, which is already saturated, and to carry out financial transactions with distant economies. The interlinkage of markets and cultures has been promoted, mainly, by the development of telecommunications, information technologies, and telematics (technology that integrates, in a single device, telecommunication resources—telephone, television, satellites, and optical fibers—and information technology—computers, *software,* and network systems), making it possible for businesses with longstanding countries to be carried out with low-cost investment.

These are the landmarks in the process of increasing these technologies: the beginning of international transmission of television via satellite, in the mid-1960s; the creation and accelerated diffusion of computers, in the 1980s, followed by the invention and propagation of *laptops, tablets,* etc.; the invention of mobile telephony and its worldwide dissemination in the 1980s and early 1990s; the revolution in digital technology with the popularization of the *Internet* in the 1990s—which, as a worldwide communication network, allows the instantaneous communication and transfer of information and data; the advent of *smartphones* in the first decade of the twenty-first century, which results from the integration of digital technology with connectivity via the Internet and cell phone; the creation of *online* social networks such as *Orkut* and *Facebook,* both from 2004, and *Twitter* from 2006.

Devices that allow quick access to information have become desired goods and seem to be more and more indispensable to meet the requirements of the new world order. It is important to emphasize that it is not only a high speed of updating information that is expected by society but also the ability to handle an abundant volume of information. This unprecedented technological development has produced an even greater acceleration in the execution of daily tasks. In the society of productivity, the time saved has been filled with more tasks and not with idleness.

Kehl (2009) establishes a relationship between the acceleration of individual and collective temporal experience, which reaches the maximum speed of instantaneousness in postmodern times, and the loss of the value of experience in current culture. This acceleration, according to the author, would be a central cultural variable for the understanding of depression in the contemporary world. If the difficulty in stopping and "doing nothing," the urgency in frantically taking advantage of idleness time and immediacy were already relevant aspects for a cultural analysis of depression in the mid-1980s (Skinner 1986), those aspects became even more critical in the present. In postmodern society, in which capitalism broadens its horizons and expands its already high productivity, technologies are developed to promote the frenetic acceleration of daily life; stopping and "doing nothing" generate, as never before, feelings of guilt, inferiority, and social inadequacy—all of which are constituents of depression.

The increase of stress in postmodern life (produced by extreme dedication to work, dependence on electronic devices, exposure to various stimuli in urban centers, among other contemporary trends) is being discussed as one of the factors possibly related to the high prevalence of depression in the present world (e.g. Kessler 1997; Whybrow 2006). Moderate Chronic Stress (MCS) is an experimental model of depression that serves as an analytical tool to understand, in a behavioral way, how the stress of contemporary life can be related to depression. We know that chronic exposure to mild stress, increasingly present in the daily life of the postmodern world, can produce anhedonia. Therefore, there are experimental data that allow us to explain how the daily stress of postmodern life can act as one of the determinants of depression culture in the present.

Hidaka (2012) presents a list of specific factors of contemporary Western culture that could explain why "in the desire to accumulate material wealth and a growing standard of living, young people have a greater risk of depression than their parents and grandparents" (p. 207). As an example of this greater risk, the author relates the case of metropolitan China, which has undergone a rapid cultural transformation in recent decades and which has presented a dramatically increased risk of depression: Chinese people born before 1966 have a 22.4 times greater chance of developing MDD than those born before 1937.

Among the aspects considered by Hidaka (2012) as specific to contemporary Western culture (and to the Eastern cultures westernized by globalization) are impoverishment of the quality of the food diet (the author presents data on correlation between obesity and depression and data on the adherence to the Mediterranean diet as a factor that diminishes the risks of depression); physical inactivity (less than the half of American adults are engaged in the recommended amount of physical exercise, there is a critical correlation between sedentary behavior and greater risk of depression); endocrine dysfunctions due to inadequate exposure to the sun (decreased exposure to sunlight and circulatory deregulation are causes of seasonal affective disorders—there is a cultural pattern of inadequate sun exposure evidenced by the modern epidemic of vitamin D deficiency); lack of sleep (data indicate that reduced sleeping hours in the average American adult and insomnia doubles the risk of developing depression) (Hidaka 2012).

Bauman (2001, 2004a, b, 2013), an important sociologist today, proposes the concept of *liquid modernity* to emphasize "fluidity," "speed," and "immediacy" as central marks of the capitalism of our times, at the time when Debord (1997a, b), a contemporary Marxist theorist who sets out to analyze the current forms of alienation, presents the concept of *spectacle* to defend that the distinctive quality of postmodern society is the intermediation of social relationships through images (Debord 1997a, b). Presenting the central ideas of these two thinkers of postmodern society can serve to begin to identify the new contingencies prevailing in the contemporary world and their relationship with the production of depression.

The central aspect of Debord's critical theory (1997a, b) is that the constant transformation of reality into spectacle, or false reality, would serve the new forms of social domination in this stage of capitalism, in which the social fabric is permeated by images (Debord 1997a, b). An example of the transformation of reality into spectacle is the Gulf War, which took place in 1991, the first war transmitted live. The existence of new technologies for broadcasting images, via satellite and with optical fibers, allowed international telejournalism networks to be created, such as *Cable News Network* (CNN), that emerged in the 1980s with the objective of presenting news 24 h a day throughout the week. CNN became famous with the outbreak of the Gulf War by providing uninterrupted coverage of the combat. Unprecedented images were captured, and television networks from all over the world bought and transmitted live the scenes of the war show. The images of missiles illuminating the city of Iraq were aired daily on television throughout the world, becoming emblematic and giving it the name of "video game war". In an era in which immediate information has become central to everyday life, CNN's instant news published worldwide by different media has proven to be crucial for the formation of a public opinion favorable to the US attack (Mancuso 2009).

What makes this war postmodern is not the use of media as an instrument of war, but the spectacularization of war, the speed of transmission of images, which reaches the maximum limit of immediacy and the scope of dissemination of information in space, which becomes practically global. In this sense, Mancuso (2009) makes an analysis of the transmission of the Gulf War from Debord's concept of spectacle (1997a, b). Therefore, the author proposes to explain in a didactic way this central concept in Debord's work:

> In this stage of the capitalist mode of production, capital has reached such a degree of accumulation that it has become detached from its own merchandise in its physical form, transforming itself into an image. In this way, everything that is not only produced, but also lived in these societies is transformed into merchandise and, therefore, can be consumed. However, the spectacle is not only the set of these images produced by the capital, but the process in which the images become the mediators of the social relations between people. Although capitalism is real as much as the society that makes it work, the spectacle transforms real life into unreality and consubstantiation in the dominant social relation model of society (Debord 1997a, b, p. 372).

The images consist, therefore, in new forms of capital and become consumer goods propagated by means of communication and mass media, whose scope has been greatly expanded by recent technological development. To understand what would be, in behavioral terms, the "spectacle society" and the "images" that mediate social relations and that constitute the dominant model of social relationships will be fundamental in analyzing the current social production of depression.

Advertising, as verbal stimulation, has always had the objective of leading the consumer to buy a certain product. This effect can be produced by means of different stimulus control operations, such as the presentation of discriminative stimuli, rules and/or establishing operations, construction of arbitrary relations of stimulus equivalence (Rakos 1993) or other types, such as those studied by the RFT (Rakos 1997). Therefore, advertising can function as an antecedent stimulation (which presents new stimuli or modifies the functions of already existing ones) that controls the consuming responses.

A first behavioral translation of what Debord (1997a) conceives as "The Society of the Spectacle" that transforms "image into consumer goods" could be a set of cultural practices mainly exerted by media and propaganda, as control agencies, which aim at establishing arbitrary relations between a given market and other reinforcers already established in modern culture (e.g., individual power, social status, superiority, and success). In this way, a certain merchandise acquires a reinforcing function, or rather, it becomes an object of consumption, not because of the attributes directly established by its use, but through transformation of function. The reinforcing function is derived, transferred from other already established reinforcers; this "symbolic function" would be the "image" that is consumed.

To understand why such a cultural practice was selected, it is worth mentioning that the consumer society derives directly from the industrial development, since, at a certain point, it became more difficult to sell the products and services than manufacture them. In a nutshell, in the consumer society the production of goods exceeds the consumption; the methods of manufacture are based on the production in series; the production in series diminishes the price of the products; the standards of consumption need to be massified to distribute the production; the people need to be induced to buying even when they are not in a state of deprivation. Thus, the companies started to use aggressive and seductive marketing strategies in order to create new needs and motivations. Part of these strategies consists of encouraging the consumer to buy according to the "image" of a certain product, in its symbolically and arbitrarily established function. As the acquisition of these products symbolized the acquisition of "social status," "power," "success," this form of consumption became central in postmodern society for individuals to feel integrated and valued socially.

If, in the first stage of capitalism, consumption was stimulated by propagating the good qualities of the products, that is, the reinforcing functions established directly by their use, then a second stage began: consumption was stimulated by arbitrarily relating the product to various social status indicators, which are quite important in a competitive and individualistic society. This was the first stage in the process of dislocation of the value of the goods of their use and of transformation of capital into image.

It happens that capitalism has advanced, and in postmodernity the consumer markets have been and are still being expanded. New technologies and products continue to be invented at an ever-increasing speed—and the market economy cannot slow down. To guarantee the survival of the new practices of the capitalist economy, the increase in the volume of production must be accompanied by an increase in the amount of consumption. Thus, new strategies of behavioral control have been combined through media and propaganda with the objective of stimulating consumption, giving rise to a second stage of the process of transformation of capital into image. The new mass culture goes on to establish and divulge that people now pay more attention to appearances, in what is new, modern, beautiful. The aesthetically sensitive and sophisticated consumer is valued and gains social status. Design and market go on to work together to induce the consumer to frequently and repeatedly buy the latest model, discarding the previous one—even if it works well, or that is, even though it has a reinforcement function directly established by its use.

In this new moment of capitalism, the desire to consume the latest model, to discard the "old" merchandise—even if it was manufactured and bought very recently—became symbolically related to "well-being," "happiness," "success," and "prosperity." A printed advertisement of an Iphone 4S illustrates well the construction of arbitrary relationships between consuming the new model of cell phone and being "fulfilled" and "happy." The picture is of a bride throwing her Iphone 4, the previous model, to the single women as if it were a bouquet. The bride has a surprise on her face and above her appear the following words *something new* (something new) and the women who are single appear to fight over the mobile phone, with the phrase *something old* above. Owning the new Iphone is related to getting married, achieving a social status, being a desired and fulfilled woman, etc. At the same time, to be with the old model is to "go backwards," to lose, to not be desired and socially valued as a woman.

In this way, the discardability of commercialism, or consumerism, became highly stimulated and symbolically established as the equivalent to a prosperous, fulfilled life, "what worked." Thus, "consuming what is newest" becomes a value of contemporary culture; a value in the sense defined by Leigland (2005) of being a reinforcer that acquires its function due to its participation in relational networks. Consuming the new and discarding the "old" becomes the new way of producing social belonging (Leigland 2005).

Postmodern subjects do not only want to have beautiful, pleasant, and amusing things because of the pleasure produced by contact with such stimuli, as Skinner analyzed (Skinner 1986). They want to consume in order to be happy, fulfilled, and socially acceptable. More than that, they want to consume because this way of life has become a way in which they think about, evaluate, and feel their value as individuals; "to have," "to possess" has become the way in which individuals identify who they are; to consume has become a question of the identity and subjectivity of the postmodern subject. It seems that here is a central variable to understanding the social production of depression today.

However, before going deeper into this issue, it is worth noting that when Debord (1997a, b) talks about the "The Society of the Spectacle," he is referring to the fact that not only the products but also what is lived in these societies, turn into merchandise to be consumed. More than that, the "spectacle" is the process by which images mediate social relations, becoming the dominant model of social relationship.

A possible behavioral analysis of what Debord (1997a, b) is discussing when referring to the "The Society of the Spectacle" is if, in the first moment, the cultural practices of the West promoted a certain lifestyle (the one analyzed by Skinner (1986), and in the second moment, when from the passage of modernity to postmodernity, cultural practices transformed the very lifestyle into spectacle (Skinner 1986). This is the spectacle that postmodern subjects exhibit to others—and are therefore applauded, or rather, reinforced with the most different demonstrations of social valuation—and desire to consume, as audience of other people lives, when these are considered the most successful. It is exactly because the cultural practices of postmodernity made it important to exhibit, demonstrate, and have the appearance, that life is lived as an ideal of this culture—hedonistic, consumerist, happy, very productive, accelerated etc.,—that the spectacle transforms real life into unreality or false realities, as Debord affirms (Debord 1997a, b).

In behavioral terms, social appreciation has become so contingent on the stories and demonstrations of life considered ideal by this culture that such stories and exhibitions of lived experiences can become modulated and, to a limited extent, distorted. According to Debord (1997a, b), the "images constructed" on one's own life and "divulged" by an individual become the mediators of social relations, or rather, they function as antecedents that control the responses of other individuals— of showing that life considered ideal is being lived. Such antecedents, because they are consistent with the elements already culturally established as synonyms of the ideal life, constitute another source of control over the behavior of other individual(s).

Thus, the accumulation of experiences consistent with the ideal of propagated life, at first by the media and now also by many individuals of this culture, increases the control and "coherence" of the propagated content. The one who goes on to "spectacularize" his own life in these terms has greater chances of producing social appreciation of different sources and, as a result, feels part of the social group. From distortions of stories and evidence of the lived reality, or rather, from the creation of spectacles as false realities for the other to watch and applaud, the postmodern subjects produce a real feeling of belonging.

In this way, the cultural practices that involve excessive control of responses by verbal antecedents (verbal governance) and for consequent of "social approval" type—the fourth and fifth practices analyzed by Skinner (1986) as producers of apathy and depression—gain even larger proportions. They become more prevalent, including the modulation and distortion of the stories as a function of the consequent social valuation, further restricting the contact with the intrinsic reinforcers that are produced by the direct exploration of contingencies and reducing, therefore, the diversity of sources of reinforcement and the behavioral variability. As a consequence, the dominant model of social relationship in this society becomes one of uninterrupted adherence to one's own image and to the image itself; of observation and scrutiny of signs that evidence that the life being lived is the good life, the happy and full life. Contemporary subjects "are subject to mass media that encourages comparison with others of higher social status, motivating the search for unreachable goals" (Geaney 2011, p. 512). Life spectacles, while distortions, transformations of real life into unreality, create the illusion that there is in fact a life with full consumer power, constant state of happiness and pleasure, continuous well-being, high productivity, and professional fulfillment.

How could the fact that this ideal of life has become an object of consumption in the West be related to high rates of depression? The British psychologist Oliver James (1998, 2007a, b, 2008) has researched this question. James's first book (1998) has as its title a question very similar to that posed by Skinner (1986)—*Britain on the Couch: Why We're Unhappier Compared with 1950, Despite Being Richer—A Treatment for the Low-serotonin Society.* Its central argument is that advanced capitalism makes money out of dissatisfaction, to the extent that it encourages individuals to relieve the feeling of discontent and unhappiness by acquiring material goods. From the author's perspective, the work of advertisers is to create false needs and, since the beginning of the 1970s, or rather, at the beginning of postmodernity, these have grown enormously. According to James (1998, 2007a, b, 2008), at the beginning of capitalism, people wanted things because they were useful; later, they started to want things to improve their social status, and now they want to avoid feeling ugly, unhealthy, etc.

James (2007a) uses the term *afluenzza*, which originated from the joining of the words *affluence* (wealth, abundance of good materials) and *influenza* (flu), to refer to a species of viral infection, socially transmitted, of obstinate persecution for possessing more and more consumer goods in search of wealth and personal satisfaction (James 2007a). Afluenzza, according to James (2007a), it is the cultural pattern of consuming obsessively; constantly comparing their financial pattern and consumer goods with those of other individuals; desiring for what one does not have and for being more (beautiful, successful, rich, happy, etc.) than what one is; to invest in "keeping up appearances" that are socially valued; to be constantly concerned with what others think of us; to believe that all human needs can be satisfied by consumption.

The "virus" would be spelled out because it feeds on itself: the media builds ideals of beauty, professional success, social relations, love, etc. The individual, in search of social valuation, modulates and distorts their story, transforming real life into unreality and contributing, thus, to the propagation of this illusory ideal; the individual compares aspects of their lives with those massively propagated in culture and invariably feels dissatisfied with not being enough. As culture teaches that needs are suppressed by consumption and that individual value is linked to wealth, success, beauty and happiness, the dissatisfied individual buys—clothes, artificial tanning, cars, aesthetic treatments, technological equipment, etc.—and the cycle repeats itself.

In synthesis, the thesis defended by James (1998, 2007a, b, 2008) is that "selfish capitalism" led to a massive increase in wealth, generated greater social inequality, and was responsible for the enormous increase in the prevalence of depression, anxiety and substance abuse. Based on the defining aspects of the concept of "selfish capitalism," James (2008) considers the main English-speaking countries (USA, Britain, Australia, Canada, New Zealand) as countries with "selfish capitalism"[2] and the continental countries of Western Europe (Denmark, Netherlands, Spain) and Japan, as relatively unselfish capitalist countries (James 2008). This would explain, according to the author, the substantial difference (practically double) in the average prevalence found in the USA and New Zealand of cases of depression, anxiety, and substance abuse (23.6%), compared with the average of continental Western European countries and Japan (11.5%).

Over a period of 9 months, James (2007b) traveled to different cities around the world (Sydney, Singapore, Moscow, Copenhagen, New York, Shanghai, etc.), where he interviewed their inhabitants and found that the "virus" of affluence is spreading

---

[2]The characteristics of "egoist capitalism" are the evaluation of business success, in large part based on the current stock prices; a strong impulse to privatize collective markets—water, gas, electricity, etc.; minimal regulations of financial and labor market services; conviction that the consumer and the market choices may supply almost all those types of human necessities.

in different cultures at different levels of richness. Furthermore, in countries with characteristics of "selfish capitalism," it was found that money, appearance (social and physical, and fame are highly valued, and these aspects are consistently correlated with mental disorders (James 2007b). The relationship between this set of values and the production of depression is also discussed by other authors (e.g., Pickett and Wilkinson 2010; Whybrow 2006; Bauman 1998).

Bauman (1998), in Postmodernity and Its Discontents, *O Mal-Estar da Pós-Modernidade,* thickens the chorus of those who identify the hyperstimulation of consumption as a new source of current human suffering. The author argues that, in postmodernity, the precocity in consuming and the hedonistic morality inflated the desires at the point of these acquiring unrealistic proportions. The disparity between desire and reality generates a constant dissatisfaction. A life centered on consumption would continually feed impossible desires and then frustrate them.

How, from the point of view of the Behavior Analysis, can these new postmodernity contingencies be a source of depression? It is possible that the postmodern culture (competitive, consumerist and hedonist) teaches its members to perceive and feel its value from the incessant comparison between its personal attributes (material goods, physical attributes, sensation of happiness, etc.) and those that compose the ideal circulating in the mass media and the spectacular discourse of individuals. However, exactly because this ideal is unreal and unreachable, individuals fall into a trap from which they can only feel unhappy, inferior, and dissatisfied with themselves.

Competitive culture teaches that the value of the individual is found in comparison with others. Thus, the individual is urged to constantly emit a relational response of comparison between his attributes and those possessed by others. However, exactly because the standard with which they compare themselves is unreal, although massively circulating (which gives a false illusion of reality), their personal attributes are, almost inevitably, "less than" the standard of a happy, good and "normal" life. As researches on transformation of consequential value via relational response of comparison demonstrate (e.g., Whelan and Barnes-Holmes 2004), once such events, in the case of personal attributes, are arbitrarily related as "less than", they will be transformed into less powerful reinforcers. As our culture establishes an equivalence relationship between "me" and "my attributes" (e.g., Hayes et al. 2012; Wilson and Soriano 2002), the loss of their reinforcing value results in the sensation of loss of individual value as a whole. Sensations of low self-esteem, incapacity, and inferiority are expected consequences. Moreover, as reinforcers lose their value, one can expect a low behavioral frequency of the behavioral classes that produce them. Thus, low inclination to act, discouragement, and apathy are predictable behavioral changes. These feelings and the low inclination to behave make up the depressed pattern.

Another factor that deserves attention is that, from the moment in which the individual value is strongly influenced by the income and power of consumption, the postmodern individual begins to devote much of his time to producing reinforcers related to material wealth and possessions. Reinforcers of another nature, such as those produced by family contact, friendship, love relationships or by other activities not related to social status, pass to control less the behavior. The low density of the reinforcement by affective contact and the restriction in the sources of reinforcement can also be critical variables in the production of depression.

Another consequence of the fact that the individual identity and value become dependent on demonstrations of consumer power is the increased effort to "keep up appearances" that are socially valued and the degree of concern about what others think of us. Therefore, postmodern individuals are considerably more dependent on a type of reinforcement which, because it is of social origin, is essentially unstable, since the reinforcement varies from moment to moment to depend on the conditions of the reinforcer agents (cf. Skinner 1965). The insecurity generated by the instability of the social reinforcement system gains more drastic results in a culture that is organized on the basis of competitive contingencies, because if the dominant logic is that having an individual value means being "better than" the others, the individuals become less likely to value the others. In competitive social relations, the density of social approval coming from the members is, by definition, low, when it exists. This is also one of the factors that must be related to the production of depression in the postmodern world, which is more competitive than ever. It is possible that, in competitive groups, individuals even control the actions of others who function as social reinforcers, but these are not explicit demonstrations of valuation. They are subtle signs of recognition that the individual has—or is—something that he wishes to have or to be, so signs of envy and jealousy become a social reinforcement, essentially, in competitive groups. In another way, the individual encounters in the social environment a low density of reinforcers and, when he does, they are of the type that does not promote approximation or cooperation. On the contrary, they increase competitiveness and make the individual less likely to be a social environment that reinforces the behavior of others. Thus, it is easy to visualize that a course of these interactions is a kind of effective social isolation, which is known to be related to depression.

In this sense, that "dense and warm" social environment described by Ariés and Duby (1990) as characteristic of premodernity has, throughout Western history, gradually become cooling and becoming rarefied. Today what we have is a social environment that is affectively cold (Ariés and Duby 1990). The warm, when it exists, is "liquid" and not "solid," ephemeral, and not dense (Bauman 2004a). The relationship of this aspect with the production of depression will be more deeply discussed ahead.

Another consequence of the advance of capitalism in its postmodern phase is the increase in social inequality (e.g., Bauman 2013; Hidaka 2012; James 2007b), an aspect related to the production of mental diseases, especially in rich and unequal countries (e.g., Pickett and Wilkinson 2010). Kate Pickett and Richard Wilkinson are researchers and professors in Social Epidemiology who investigate the statistical relationship between levels of social inequality and the prevalence of mental disorders. Pickett and Wilkinson (2010) demonstrate a strong relationship between the level of social inequality in rich countries and the percentage of the population with mental illness (Pickett and Wilkinson 2010). Using as a source of data, the *World Mental Health Survey* organized by the WHO, the authors verify that, in Germany, Italy, Japan, and Spain (developed countries with less social inequality), less than 1 in 10 individuals had some type of mental illness in the year prior to the research; In Australia, Canada, New Zealand, and the UK (developed countries with greater social inequality), the rate found was higher—more than one in every five individuals; in the USA (a developed country with greater social inequality), the highest rate—more than one in every four individuals—was evident. The relationship between some subtypes of mental illness and social inequality was also examined. The authors identify a correlation between mood disorders (between them, depression) and social inequality, although not as strong as that found for anxiety disorders, impulse, and addiction disorders. Pickett and Wilkinson (2010) conclude that social inequality is a source of mental illness and suffering that has received less attention than it should.

> Our impression is that greater inequality increases the state of competition and insecurity. Internationally and among the 50 states of the United States, income inequality is strongly related to low levels of confidence, lesser community life and increased violence. Mental health is deeply influenced by the quality and adequacy of social relations and all these measures suggest that both are affected by inequality (Pickett and Wilkinson 2010, p. 427).

Hidaka (2012) conducted a study on the correlation between social inequality and depression (Hidaka 2012). Like Pickett and Wilkinson (2010), based on the data from the *World Mental Health Survey*, but correlates the data with *Gini coefficient* data (a measure of social inequality that varies from 0 to 1, with 1 being the most unequal) from various countries. The author finds a strong correlation between social inequality and depression risk. Especially in developed countries, the greater the social inequality, the greater the prevalence of depression, as illustrated in Fig. 3.1.

According to Hidaka (2012), the establishment of a major depressive episode often coincides with a stressful life event (Hidaka 2012). Thus, a more unequal social environment could contribute to the growth of depression rates, since it is constituted by more frequent and severe social adversities, such as: increasing competitiveness (e.g.,

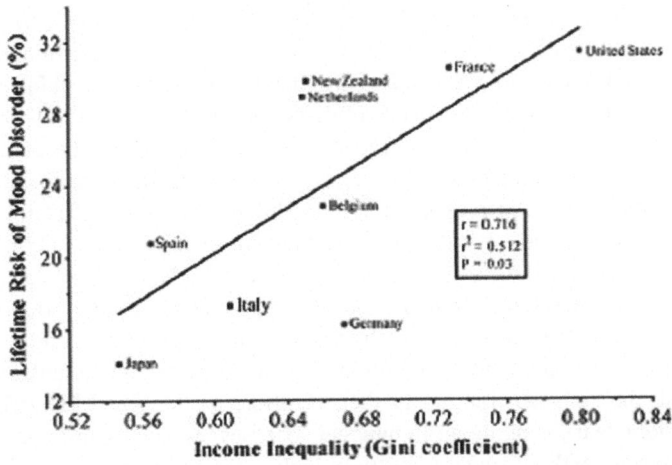

Fig. 3.1 Correlation between wage inequality and risk of depression throughout life (reproduced from Hidaka 2012)

workers compete for jobs now on a global scale); more threatened social contacts; bigger social isolation; increased chances of social failure; and low social support. Perhaps for this reason, higher rates of depression are found in Mexicans born in the USA compared with Mexican immigrants (Vega et al. 2004). It is interesting to note that Japan (a country with a lower prevalence of depression), although it has a highly modernized and capitalist society, has little social inequality and a culture that emphasizes collectivism over individualism. These two factors should add to the social environment protection against the development of depression. It is possible that social inequality impacts, in different ways, the quality of social relations in the sense of making individuals more vulnerable to depression. The following is a possible behavioral interpretation of the relationship between social inequality and depression.

Those who possess a high income, with fear of losing their high position in the social hierarchy, are incessantly looking for more and more material wealth. The excess of behavior controlled by maintaining and expanding economic power is accompanied by a low frequency of behaviors related to the establishment and cultivation of relationships with family and friends, resulting in a financially rich life, yet effectively poor. Feelings of loneliness, sadness, and emptiness are more than expected. The competitive social contingencies overlap, in this way, the existence of community and cooperative social contingencies and, with this, the production of a specific type of feeling of well-being and social belonging.

This part of the population also suffers from the constant fear of violence from those who have less. The greater the social inequality, the greater the chances of theft, robbery, kidnapping, murder, etc. Small daily signs of the possible occurrence of adverse events of this order possibly function as varied chronic stressors and produce anhedonia (Moderate Chronic Stress, as discussed above, is one of the experimental models for depression). Nevertheless, the highest prevalence of depression in the 12 months prior to the survey is found in São Paulo, Brazil, higher even than that found in 18 countries (Kessler and Bromet 2013; Kessler and Üstün 2008). Current data (Bichir et al. 2012) reveal the high rates of inequality and social vulnerability in São Paulo and, if related to the analysis carried out by Pickett and Wilkinson (2010), help to understand the high prevalence of depression found in this city.

Those with average incomes suffer from chronic dissatisfaction because they are forced to continually compare themselves with those at the top of the social ranking; they are condemned to consider their unsuccessfulness with certain bitterness and as proof of their lesser worth as individuals. Such result seems even more cruel when it is considered that this same society imposes and values a highly accelerated rhythm of productivity. Therefore, the individual feels at same time exhaustion and lack of energy, because they work too much, and a feeling of emptiness and incapacity, because they "never get there." There is also the uncertainty and dissatisfaction that comes with the real vulnerability of their positions in the social hierarchy; those who have jobs fear losing them. In unequal societies, especially in those of developing countries (without social security policies), losing income means becoming economically and socially unprotected; it means social defeat. Research shows that unemployment and depression are highly related (e.g., Kessler 2012; Lépine and

Briley 2011)—since losing income means losing access to many material and social supporters, it is not difficult to understand why. Not only that individuals from the so-called "middle class" are also victims of exposure to chronic daily stressors in unequal and violent societies. It is no exaggeration to say that this segment of the population (larger in terms of numbers than the richest segment) has fewer resources to buy ways to reduce the contact with such daily stressors (armored cars, security houses, high walls, alarm systems, etc.), thus increasing their exposure to this source of anhedonia.

Those who have low income or almost none at all are those who suffer from the most varied forms of social exclusion—poor, marginalized, racially discriminated, ethnic minorities, illegal immigrants, etc.,—and they live the multiple unfolding of a state of abandonment and brutal social isolation. Bauman (2013) analyzes social inequality as a product of our "liquid-modern" world and the disadvantaged people as "collateral damage" of a profit-oriented and consumption-oriented society; they are "strangers inside," deprived of the rights enjoyed by other members of the social order (Bauman 2013). It is not by chance that Os et al. (2010) discovered that growth in the urban environment and belonging in minority groups are environmental factors highly related to the development of schizophrenia (Os et al. 2010). In certain social minority groups, the risk of presenting schizophrenic symptoms may be five times greater. The authors discuss how the appearance of symptoms may be an effect of chronic social adversities, as a result of marginalization and social defeat.

The absence of conditions (i.e., work) to produce material reinforcers that guarantee subsistence, the very low density of social reinforcement due to social exclusion, and the abundance of chronic social problems (in the form of social deprivation and even punishment) are clearly aspects that produce depression. Added are two other aspects to these factors: (1) the absence of positively consequential responses classes by society, to the extent that the social fabric considers them as inexistent (except for the constant evil and threat that they represent) and (2) a state of social abandonment produced by contact with uncontrollable aggressive stimuli. In Bauman's (2013) words:

> The idea of "subclass" suggests that there is no function to be performed (as in the case of the "working" or "professional" classes), nor a position occupied in the social sphere (as in the case of the "low", "medium" or "high" classes). The only meaning that the term "subclasse" has is *to be outside* of any significant classification, oriented to the position and function. The "subclass" may be "within", but clearly it is not "of" society: it does not contribute at all that society needs to obtain its survival and well-being; in fact, society would be better off without it. The condition of the "subclass", as suggested by the name attributed to it, is that of "internal emigrants", or "illegal immigrants", "outsiders" - removed from the rights enjoyed by recognized and approved members of society; in short, a foreign body that is not counted among the "natural" and indispensable parts of the social organism. Something not different from a cancerous tumor, the most effective treatment is its removal, or at least its forced, induced and planned confinement and/or remission (Bauman 2013, p. 10).

Bauman (2013) analyzes the selective affinity between the increase in social inequality and the expansion of the volume of "collateral damage" and highlights the following characteristics as marks of contemporaneity: indifference in relation to others; hypertrophy of subjectivity; decline of ethical judgment in human relations;

tendency of authorities to exempt themselves from in face of exclusion, considering it a necessary evil.

Various contemporary authors present writings that are consistent with Bauman's diagnosis (2013), pointing to the loss of references of collective projects as emblems of post-modernity, intensifying the process of individualization, lessening belonging to social groups, detaching from original cultural circles (including the family), which generates immigration and deterritorialization accompanied by greater chances of exclusion and social abandonment (e.g., Murcia 2006; Fuentes and Quiroga 2005) and "narcissism as a cultural phenomenon" (e.g., Lasch 1983).

In previous books, Bauman (2001, 2004b) had already discussed how the dissolutions in the affective and social bonds became a central issue in the sphere of individual and collective life in "liquid modernity." This concept is proposed by the author to describe social transformations by which contemporary society passes in all spheres: public and private life, human relations, the world of work, the state, and social institutions. The concept is presented

> not that it seems an attempt to offer "fluidity" as the main metaphor for the present situation of the modern era... The extraordinary mobility of fluids is what associates them with the idea of "lightness"... We associate "lightness" or "absence of weight" with mobility and inconstancy: we know in practice that the lighter we travel, the easier and faster we move (Bauman 2001, p. 8).

According to Bauman (2001), current capitalism is infinitely faster, more dynamic, "fluid," "light," "liquid" than that which existed until the 1970s. Since then, we have entered a new era, "a new era in many ways, in the history of modernity" (Bauman 2001, p. 9). In the collective sphere, the solids that are melting in this moment of fluid modernity are those that interweave individual choices in projects and collective actions, while in the individual sphere they are those that interweave individuals in social relationships that are more durable and resistant to frustration. The logic of consumption, because it is highly pervasive, has penetrated the sphere of intimate social relationships and has conferred on the relationship with the other market players a sense of discardability and ephemerality (Bauman 2001, 2004a). In liquid modernity, there is no compromise with the idea of permanence and durability. Contemporary individuals live in a paradox: at the same time that they are looking for *Liquid Love* (Bauman 2004a)—affective detachment, preservation of freedom and uncommitting in relationships—they complain of loneliness and isolation. The supposed sensation of freedom brings, on its flip side, the evidence of the lack of effective abandonment in which the "modern-liquid" individuals find themselves.

Other authors also identify as markers of contemporary subjectivity: coldness in relationships, distant effectiveness, preservation of individual interests over collective interests (e.g., Pérez-Alvaréz 2003); indifference in relation to others, and ethics of individual well-being (e.g., Lasch 1983; Murcia 2006). Depression, as a set of symptoms that involves loneliness, social isolation, feeling of lack of affectivity, is one of the costs of a life with low density of affection. The data on the strong relationship between depression and the end of effective relationship (e.g., Lépine and Briley 2011; Bromet et al. 2011) seem to support this assertion.

As a result, we have an individualized and privatized version of modernity, and the weight of the pattern and responsibility for failure falls mainly on the shoulders of individuals. This has led to the liquidation of dependency and interaction patterns. They are now malleable to a point that past generations did not experience and could not imagine (Bauman 2004a, p. 14).

One change in the pattern of social interaction that is also seen as defining post-modern sociability is the transformation of youth and adolescence as ideas of culture; everyone wants to be young and not adult, as they were at the beginning of the nine-teenth century. The USA transformed the individuals who live in the long "social moratorium" of adolescence in potential consumers. The construction of youth as an ideal of culture has been rapidly disseminated in the capitalist world (Kehl 2004). This change seems also fundamental in understanding the production of depression today. The basis of the argument is launched by Kehl (2004):

> On the one hand, the association between youth and consumption favored the flourishing of a highly hedonistic adolescent culture. The adolescent of the last decades of the 20th century stopped being a big, unassigned and inhibited child, with no sense of shame and antisocial habits, to become the model of beauty, freedom and sensuality for all the other age groups. The postmodern adolescent enjoys all the freedoms of adult life, but he is spared almost all the responsibilities (pp. 46–47).

As the author explains in this passage, youth and adolescence stopped being arbi-trarily related to socially devalued aspects and started, in post-modernity, to be related to beauty, freedom, pleasure and sensuality. So that symbolic relationship contributed to the development of a consumerist, highly hedonistic culture. Hence, evidence of beauty, pleasure, contentment, and joviality have been built up as derived positive reinforcers, while sadness, laziness, low energy sensation, and aging have been built up as derived negative reinforcers. These are the main trends of postmodernity: the cult of the body and culture *fitness* (Lasch 1983); investments in the conservation of signs of youth, beauty, and feminine leanness (Raphael and Lacey 1992); biotechno-logical development and consumption of cosmetics (including a cosmetic psychiatry) to preserve youth, maximize happiness, avoid aging and any type of suffering (Pardo and Pérez-Álvarez 2007); avoidance of suffering that is inherent in life—an aspect identified by Skinner (1986) and widely discussed today (Harris 2007; Hayes et al. 2012; Kehl 2004; Pardo and Pérez-Álvarez 2007; Wilson and Soriano 2002). In this regard, the greater social demands on women than on men, when it comes to the conservation of signs of beauty and youth, together with the accumulation of social roles, are considered by some authors as cultural determinants of the greater preva-lence of some psychopathologies in women than men, such as anorexia (e.g., Raphael and Lacey 1992) and depression (e.g., Lafrance 2009).

Part of the dominant discourse in the hedonistic culture that venerates consump-tion, youth, beauty, and happiness as an ideal of life, is the promotion of equiv-alence relations between "happiness" and "normality." In this culture, "suffering" is synonymous with "abnormality." Life is, therefore, a perpetual state of youthful euphoria and suffering, something to be avoided once it means not being normal (Harris 2007; Kehl 2009; Wilson and Soriano 2002). This is, therefore, another way in which "happiness" becomes a powerful social value through the transference of function. Also, through the transference of function "sadness" acquires an aversive value, potentialized by contemporary culture.

What is more surprising is that the same culture that reproduces a hegemonic discourse eminently *antidepressant,* it also produces, according to the numbers shown by epidemiological research, an alarming rate of depression. How do these two apparently contrary trends relate to each other?

According to some authors (e.g., Geaney 2011; Pardo and Pérez-Álvarez 2007; Pessotti 2001), the frenetic search for happiness has changed the "sensibility" of contemporary individuals, making them less resilient to life issues that were once not felt as signs of "problems" of mental sickness. The prevailing idea that the natural human condition is one of "perpetual euphoria" produced in postmodern individuals, an intolerance before any sign of sadness, frustration, or dissatisfaction.

Pessotti (2001), a historian on madness, denounces the fact that the times have transformed everyday problems into diagnostic categories and that the diagnosis of depression has become "fashionable." In the following section, he describes this change and indicates possible cultural determinants:

> The depression, today, taken by itself, as a disease or pathology is a very frequent diagnosis. There would even be an epidemic of depression that would devastate men. What there is, in fact, is an epidemic of such diagnoses, and this one has aspects of guilt. Depression is a fashionable thing. Firstly, because the diagnosis has dispensed with the delayed aetiological investigations (*time is money*); secondly, because the course of the eventual disease lost interest in favor of the pre-established constellation of symptoms…

> Discouragement, a feeling of incompetence or failure, pressure for the future, disinterest in new activities when one is preoccupied with something, these own worries, disturbances of sound or appetite or sexual efficiency are secular and everyday problems that in the past were called "hard life". Today, they are called "depressive disorders", in our manuals. Colloquially, even in the clinical environment, they are called depression. Like in the repetitive investments of the "media" and of the advertising, of the pharmaceutical industry.

> Finding a name for suffering or love reduces anxiety, it is known. If this name covers a great variety of sufferings and pressures, they are somehow framed or confronted when they receive a name. Therefore, considering oneself depressed is a way to reduce anxieties. And to open up a lot of further inquiries about oneself, which are not always pleasant. Labeling or being labeled is easy. This is one of the reasons why depression is so popular.

> Another is the hygienic influence of the "media", to urge the need to be always perfectly livers, of body and mind. Transforming any sensation of abnormality into symptoms of weakness and inferiority in such a way that health passes to imply some form of hypochondria, or rather, mental health implies mental weakness. With the consequent search of a sign and a way of cure, that restores the sensation of being well, of being normal (Pessotti 2001, pp. 53–54).

Several other authors, among them psychologists, pharmacologists, and psychiatrists, have identified and analyzed a change in the cultural practice of establishing diagnostic criteria for depression. On the basis of this debate, there is an extensive discussion on: the definition of normality versus abnormality (cf. Geaney 2011; Maj 2011); depression as a biological entity or a social-historical construction; the role of the pharmacological industry and the media in the construction and dissemination of a biological notion of depression; among other aspects (cf. Burns 2013; Geaney 2011; Pardo and Pérez-Álvarez 2007).

Analyzing the vast literature that discusses changes in the cultural practices of diagnosing and treating depression is beyond the scope of this book. However, it is important to mention that this aspect certainly figures as a central theme for a more comprehensive understanding of the discussion on cultural determinants of depression. An example of the current status of the topic is the launch, in 2013, of DSM-5 (American Psychiatric Association 2013). While the DSM-IV had a norm that guides the exclusion of the diagnosis of MDD in case the depressive symptoms are presented by a person who is in mourning for up to two months, in the new DSM-5 the exception to mourning was withdrawn. Thus, a person who is mourning for at least two weeks can now be diagnosed with depression. In the place of the rule, there are two notes asking the doctors to be cautious when making the diagnosis in cases like this. If, in fact, as Pessotti (2001) states, our culture is currently suffering from an epidemic of depression, the reduction of the limit for such diagnosis proposed by DSM-5 will aggravate the epidemic. Considering sadness or depressed mood as abnormal responses to loss can be considered "an attack of cultural panic" (Geaney 2011) and may have serious consequences, such as unnecessary medicalization and the construction of an understanding even more intolerant of the suffering inherent to life.

In conclusion, part I of this book had as its objective to offer a behavioral analysis of the sociocultural factors related to the production of depression today, based on the reflections of philosophers, social scientists, psychiatrists, and psychologists about postmodernity as well as on the interpretative and experimental models of depression that exist in the Behavior Analysis.

Given that the social risk factors for mental illness and depressive development seem to be inherent in the postmodern society, part II of this book aims to present the panorama of intervention in the area, especially focusing on innovative programs based on scientific evidence for the prevention of depression and the promotion of mental health. The need to rethink intervention strategies will be discussed, leading the reader to understand that actions aimed at reducing risk factors on a large scale are important as well as the development of social protection factors and social and emotional skills in individuals and communities.

References

American Psychiatric Association. (2013). *Diagnostic and statistical manual of mental disorders: DSM-5*. Arlington: American Psychiatric Publishing.

Ariely, D., Kamenica, E., & Prelec, D. (2008). Man's search for meaning: The case of Legos. *Journal of Economic Behavior & Organization, 67*, 671–677.

Ariés, P. (1981), *Social history of the child and the family* (2nd ed.) (Flaksman, D. Trans.) Guanabara, Rio de Janeiro, RJ.

Ariés, P., & Duby, E. (1990). *History of private life: From feudal Europe to the Renaissance*. São Paulo, SP: Companhia das Letras.

Bauman. (1998). *Or being in bad shape after the modern age* (Gama, M. and Gama, C. M. Trans.). Rio de Janeiro, RJ: Zahar.

Bauman, Z. (2001). *Liquid modernity* (Dentzien, Fr. Trans.). Rio de Janeiro, RJ: Jorge Zahar.
Bauman, Z. (2004a). *Liquid love: On the fragility of human beings* (Medeiros, C.A. Trans.). Rio de Janeiro, RJ: Jorge Zahar.
Bauman, Z. (2004b). *Identity: Interview with Benedetto Vecchi* (Medeiros, C. A. Trans.). Rio de Janeiro, RJ: Jorge Zahar.
Bauman, Z. (2013). *Give us colaterais: Sociais numa era global inequalities* (Medeiros, C.A. Trans). Rio de Janeiro, RJ: Jorge Zahar.
Bichir, R., Castello, G., & Marques, E. C. L. (2012). Social networks and social vulnerability in São Paulo and Salvador. *USP Magazine, 92,* 32–45.
Bromet, E., Andrade, L. H., Hwang, I., Sampson, N. A., Alonso, J., Girolamo, G., et al. (2011). Cross-national epidemiology of DSM-IV major depressive episode. *BMC Medicine, 9,* 90.
Bruckner, P. (1996). *A tentação da inocência.* Lisbon: Europe-America.
Burns, C. (2013), Are mental illnesses such as PMS and depression culturally determined? *The Guardian.* Retrieved from m.guardian.co.uk/science/blog/2013/may/20/mental-illnesses-depression-pms-culturally-determined.
Debord, G. (1997a). *The society of the spectacle* (Abreu, E. S. Trans.). Rio de Janeiro: Contraponto.
Debord, G. (1997b). Comentários sobre a sociedade do espetáculo. In G. Debord (Ed.), *The entertainment society* (Abreu, E. S. Trans.) (pp. 165–237). Rio de Janeiro, RJ: Contraponto.
Elias, N. (1990). *O processo civilizador: Uma história dos costumes* (Jungmann, R. Trad.). Rio de Janeiro, RJ: Jorge Zahar (Original work published in 1939).
Elias, N. (1994). *A sociedade dos indivíduos* (Ribeiro, V. Trans.). Rio de Janeiro, RJ: Jorge Zahar (Original work published in 1939).
Ferreira, D. C., & Tourinho, E. Z. (2011). Relations between depression and cultural contingencies in modern societies: Analytical and behavioural interpretation. *Brazilian Journal of Behavioral and Cognitive Therapy, 13,* 20–36.
Fuentes, J. B., & Quiroga, E. (2005). The relevance of a cultural approach to personality disorders. *Psicothema, 17,* 422–429.
Geaney, D. P. (2011). Depression: A cultural panic attack. *The British Journal of Psychiatry, 199,* 512.
Harris, R. (2007). *The happiness trap: Stop struggling, start living.* Wollombi: Exisle Publishing.
Hayes, S. C., Strosahl, K., & Wilson, K. (2012). *Acceptance and commitment therapy: The process and practice of mindful change* (2nd ed.). New York, NY: Guilford Press.
Hidaka, (2012). Depression as a disease of modernity: Explanations for increasing prevalence. *Journal of Affective Disorders, 140,* 205–214.
James, O. W. (1998). *Britain on the couch: Why we're unhappier compared with 1950, despite being richer.* London: Arrow.
James, O. W. (2007a). *Affluenza.* London: Vermillion.
James, O. W. (2007b). Selfish capitalist. *The Psychologist, 20,* 426–428.
James, O. W. (2008). *The selfish capitalist: Origins of affluenza.* London: Vermillion.
Kehl, M. R. (2009). *The time and the dog: The current state of the depressions.* São Paulo, SP: Boitempo.
Kehl, M. R. (2004). Youth as a symptom of culture. In R. Novaes & P. Vannuchi (Eds.), *Youth and society: Work, education, culture and participation* (pp. 89–129). São Paulo, SP: Fundação Perseu Abramo.
Kessler, R. C. (1997). The effects of stressful life events on depression. *Annual Review of Psychology, 48,* 191–214.
Kessler, R. C. (2012). The costs of depression. *Psychiatric Clinics of North America, 35,* 1–14.
Kessler, R. C., & Bromet, E. J. (2013). The epidemiology of depression across cultures. *Annual Review of Public Health, 34,* 119–138.
Kessler, R. C., & Üstün, T. B. (2008). *The WHO world mental health surveys: Global perspectives on the epidemiology of mental disorders.* New York, NY: Cambridge University Press.
Lafrance, M. N. (2009). *Women and depression: Recovery and resistance.* London: Routledge.

Lasch, C. (1983). *A cultura do narcisismo: A vida americana numa era de esperanças em declínio* (Pavaneli, E. Trans.). Rio de Janeiro, RJ: Imago.

Leigland, S. (2005). Variables of which values are a function. *The Behavior Analyst, 28,* 133–142.

Lépine, J. P., & Briley, (2011). The increasing burden of depression. *Neuropsychiatric Disease and Treatment, 7,* 3–7.

Maj, M. (2011). Author's reply. *The British Journal of Psychiatry, 199,* 513.

Mancuso, A. P. (2009). A war as spectacle: A reflection on the military conflicts in post-modernity. *Human Sciences Magazine, 43,* 369–382.

McLuhan, M., & Fiore, Q. (1969). *The way is a message* (Martins, I. P. Trans.). Rio de Janeiro, RJ: Record.

Murcia, M. F. (2006). Social changes and postmodern personality disorders. *Roles of the Psychologist, 27,* 104–115.

Norton, M., Ariely, D., & Mochon, D. (2012). The IKEA effect: When labor leads to love. *Journal of Consumer Psychology, 22,* 453–460.

Os, J. V., Kenis, G., & Rutten, B. P. F. (2010). The environment and schizophrenia. *Nature, 468,* 203–212.

Pardo, H. G., & Pérez-Álvarez, M. (2007). *The invention of mental disorders: Listening to the drug or the patient?* Madrid: Alianza Editorial.

Pérez-Alvaréz, M. (2003). The schizoid personality of our time. *International Journal of Psychology and Psychological Therapy, 3,* 181–194.

Pessotti, I. (2001). Depressão: Tradição e moda. In H. J. Guilhardi, M. B. B. P. Madi, P. P. Queiroz, & M. C. Scoz (Eds.), *On behavior and cognition: Vol. 7. Exposing variability* (pp. 47–55). Santo André, SP: ESETec.

Pickett, K. E., & Wilkinson, R. G. (2010). Inequality: An under acknowledged source of mental illness and distress. *The British Journal of Psychiatry, 197,* 426–428.

Rakos, R. (1993). Propaganda as stimulus control: The case of the Iraqi invasion of Kuwait. *Behavior and Social Issues, 1,* 35–62.

Rakos, R. (1997). Corporate control of media and propaganda: A behavior analysis. In P. A. Lamal (Ed.), *Cultural contingencies: Behavior analytic perspectives on cultural practices* (pp. 237–267). London: Praeger.

Raphael, F. J., & Lacey, J. H. (1992). Sociocultural aspects of eating disorders. *Annals of Medicine, 24,* 293–296.

Ricouer, P. (1975). *As culturas e o tempo.* São Paulo, SP: EDUSP.

Sennett, R. (1988). *O declínio do homem público: As tiranias da intimidade* (Watanabe, L. A. Trans.). São Paulo, SP: Companhia das Letras.

Skinner, B. F. (1965). *Science and human behavior.* New York, NY: Free Press (Original work published in 1953).

Skinner, B. F. (1986). What is wrong with daily life in the Western world? *American Psychologist, 41,* 568–574.

Tourinho, E. Z. (2009). *Subjectivity and behavioural relationships.* São Paulo, SP: Paradigm.

Vega, W. A., Sribney, W. M., Aguilar-Gaxiola, S., & Kolody, B. (2004). 12-month prevalence of DSM-III-R psychiatric disorders among Mexican Americans: Nativity, social assimilation, and age determinants. *The Journal of Nervous and Mental Disease, 192,* 532.

Wilson, K. G., & Soriano, M. C. L. (2002). *Acceptance and commitment therapy (ACT): A values-oriented behavioral treatment.* Madrid: Ediciones Pirámide.

Whelan, R., & Barnes-Holmes, D. (2004). The transformation of consequential functions in accordance with the relational frames of same and opposite. *Journal of the Experimental Analysis of Behavior, 82,* 177–195.

Whybrow, P. C. (2006). *American mania: When more is not enough.* New York, NY: WW Norton.

Index